The brain basis of emerging literacy and numeracy skills
Longitudinal neuroimaging evidence from
kindergarten to primary school

Impressum

Max Planck Institute for Human Cognitive and Brain Sciences, 2019

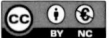

Diese Arbeit ist unter folgender Creative Commons-Lizenz lizenziert:
http://creativecommons.org/licenses/by-nc/3.0

Titelbild: © Ulrike Kuhl, 2019

Druck: DRUCKEREI Ehnert & Blankenburg GmbH, Leipzig

ISBN 978-3-941504-87-5

The brain basis of emerging literacy and numeracy skills

Longitudinal neuroimaging evidence from kindergarten
to primary school

Der Fakultät für Lebenswissenschaften

der Universität Leipzig

eingereichte

DISSERTATION

zur Erlangung des akademischen Grades

Doctor rerum naturalium

Dr. rer. nat.

vorgelegt

von Ulrike Kuhl, M.Sc.

geboren am 19. Februar 1990 in Löningen

Dekan:

Prof. Dr. Tilo Pompe

Gutachter:

Prof. Dr. Angela D. Friederici

Prof. Dr. Elke van der Meer

Tag der Verteidigung: Leipzig, den 01.10.2019

BIBLIOGRAPHISCHE DARSTELLUNG

Ulrike Kuhl

The brain basis of emerging literacy and numeracy skills —

Longitudinal neuroimaging evidence from kindergarten to primary school

Fakultät für Lebenswissenschaften

Universität Leipzig

Dissertation

217 Seiten, 440 Literaturangaben, 22 Abbildungen, 5 Tabellen

Effective literacy and numeracy skills are cornerstones of academic achievement and participation in today's digital society. Reading, writing and arithmetic problem solving are not innate but mostly learned explicitly. However, not all individuals acquire these skills with the same ease, with some showing specific learning deficits. While a large body of research identified relevant areas for literacy and numeracy processing in older children and adults, the exact nature of early pre-school correlates of typical and atypical development remains elusive. Here, structure of grey matter, whiter matter and coherence of functional circuits were investigated in children assessed longitudinally from kindergarten to the end of second grade via structural and resting-state functional magnetic resonance imaging. In the first study, children were classified as dyslexic and typically developing individuals based on their performance on standardised, age-normed reading and spelling tests. The results suggest that dyslexia reveals itself at the neural level well before children are able to read in terms of confined cortical malformation and faulty cross-talk within the speech processing system. Secondly, grey matter plasticity and its relationship with mathematical attainment in typically developing children was assessed longitudinally. The findings point to a key role of parietal, temporal and frontal cortical surface plasticity as the neurobiological foundation for successful mathematical learning in the first years of school. Relating neuroplastic correlates with typical and atypical development of literacy and numeracy skills, the findings are discussed in the light of theories of developmental dyslexia and mathematical learning.

The brain basis of emerging literacy and numeracy skills

Longitudinal neuroimaging evidence
from kindergarten to primary school

*"Literacy unlocks the door to learning throughout the life [...] and opens
the way for democratic participation and active citizenship."*
Kofi Annan, Secretary-General of the United Nations 1997–2006

*"The study of mathematics, like the Nile, begins in minuteness
but ends in magnificence."*
Charles Caleb Colton, English cleric, writer and collector

ACKNOWLEDGEMENTS

Along the winding path that lead to completion of this thesis, I have been tremendously fortunate to experience the support and encouragement of people without whom this work would not have been possible.

Firstly, I would like to express my sincere gratitude to Prof. Angela D. Friederici for her guidance and supervision, providing me with incredible research opportunities and invaluable feedback along this remarkable journey. Further, I would like to thank Prof. Angela D. Friederici and Prof. Elke van der Meer for accepting and assessing this thesis.

I owe special thanks to Dr Michael A. Skeide, who trusted my abilities, supported me when necessary and shared his expert advice, fostering my intellectual growth.

I would further like to thank my colleagues from the Department of Neuropsychology of the Max Planck Institute for Human Cognitive and Brain Sciences. I am indebted to everyone involved in the LEGASCREEN project. Dr Jan Schreiber deserves particular mention for teaching me all I know about diffusion–weighted imaging processing. Kerstin Flake, Andrea Gast–Sandman and Heike Schmidt–Duderstedt provided invaluable help with figure and document design. My thanks and appreciation go to those how grew from good colleagues into beloved friends: Clara Kühn, Clara Ekerdt, Caroline Beese, Nestor Israel Zaragoza-Jimenez, Leon Kroczek—thank you for the otterly good support that helped me persevere with this work. To Prof. Hyeon-Ae Jeon, Dr Charlotte Grosse Wiesmann, Dr Tomás Goucha, Mariella Paul, Helyne Adamson, and Patrick Trettenbrein: I thank you for your open ears and fruitful discussions. You were always there to share ideas and experiences. Furthermore, I am indebted to the children and their parents who participated in our study.

I am grateful to my family, who have provided me with tremendous moral and emotional support. Without you, I would not have come this far. I particularly wish to express my deepest gratitude to my parents, Ruth and Dieter Kuhl, for their love, guidance and encouragement. You inspire me to strive to achieve my goals, even if times are not always easy. Last—but by no means least—I would like to thank Frank, my significant other ($p < 0.001$, corrected). You are the one who keeps me up when life is trying to get me down.

CONTENTS

LIST OF FIGURES

LIST OF TABLES

LIST OF ACRONYMS

AUC	Area under the receiver operator characteristic curve
BOLD	Blood oxygenation level dependent
CF	Cortical folding complexity
CSF	Cerebrospinal fluid
CT	Cortical thickness
DD	Developmental dyslexia
DLPFC	Dorso-lateral prefrontal cortex
dMRI	Diffusion–weighted magnetic resonance imaging
EEG	Electroencephalography
FA	Fractional anisotropy
fALFF	Fractional amplitude of low frequency fluctuations
FD	Framewise displacement
fMRI	Functional magnetic resonance imaging
FOV	Field of view
FWHM	Full width at half maximum
GI	Gyrification index
GM	Grey matter
GMV	Grey matter volume
IC	Inferior colliculus
IPS	Intraparietal sulcus
LGN	Lateral geniculate nucleus

LQ	Laterality quotient
MD	Mean diffusivity
MFG	Middle frontal gyrus
MGB	Medial geniculate body
MNI	Montreal Neurological Institute
MP2RAGE	Magnetisation-prepared 2 rapid acquisition gradient echo
MRI	Magnetic resonance imaging
MTL	Medial temporal lobe
NMR	Nuclear Magnetic Resonance
PA	Phonological awareness
PFC	Prefrontal cortex
PPC	Posterior parietal cortex
RAN	Rapid automatised naming
ReHo	Regional homogeneity
RF	Radiofrequency
ROI	Region of interest
rsfMRI	Resting-state functional magnetic resonance imaging
SBM	Surface–based morphometry
SD	Sulcus depth
SPL	Superior parietal lobe
T_1	T_1-weighted
T_2^*	T_2^*-weighted
TE	Echo time
TR	Repetition time
VBM	Voxel–based morphometry
VTOC	Ventral temporal-occipital cortex

VWFA   Visual word form area

WM   White matter

CHAPTER 1

INTRODUCTION

In virtually all aspects of daily life, humans engage with written language and quantitative information. Whenever we communicate via text on a mobile device, critically scrutinise information provided in graphs or diagrams, or engage in financial transactions, we rely on effective literacy and numeracy skills. Therefore, these abilities are not just cornerstones of a sound education, but also of active participation in today's society.

Without a foundation of reliable early literacy and numeracy abilities, however, individuals struggle in daily life and fail to develop more complex, high level skills (Geary, 2011). In fact, school-entry math and reading performance rank among the most reliable predictors of later academic achievement (Duncan et al., 2007), and are thus crucial prerequisites for professional success in life.

Importantly, abilities such as reading, writing and complex arithmetic are not innate but cultural inventions that are typically learned explicitly. When acquiring literacy, one learns to link visually perceived symbols to auditory representations of language, relying on pre-existing sensory skills (Lachmann & van Leeuwen, 2014). Similarly, while prelinguistic infants as young as six months of age show a sense for magnitudes (F. Xu & Spelke, 2000), the ability to perform exact symbolic arithmetic requires formal instruction (Barth, La Mont, Lipton, & Spelke, 2005). For both literacy and mathematical abilities, developing competence involves teaching and effortful training.

Intriguingly, not all individuals acquire these skills with the same ease (M. Brown et al., 2003; Cockcroft, 1982). Even worse, some children suffer from specific impairment in literacy or maths learning. For instance, individuals suffering from developmental dyslexia (DD) struggle severely to become literate. Thereby, dyslexic children get increasingly left behind with every year in school, placing them at an educational disadvantage throughout life. Consequences not only include lasting negative effects on the affected person's mental health, such as anxiety, depression and even suicidal tendencies (Klassen, Tze, & Hannok, 2013), but affected individuals also have a greatly increased risk of criminal convictions (Alm & Andersson, 1997; Elbeheri, Everatt, & Al Malki, 2009). In this way, the failure to master basic literacy skills also constitutes a burden on society in terms of costs to the education, health and criminal justice systems (Gross, 2009).

What are the neural origins of specific differences in such complex cognitive abilities? Why do some individuals struggle with mastering these cultural inventions we impose on the brain? Considering these questions is of vital importance: A comprehensive understanding of the emergence of complex cognitive abilities and their developmental trajectories could pave the way for effective learning environments, early screening for timely identification of deficits and individualised programmes catering to the specific needs of impaired children (Butterworth & Kovas, 2013). Therefore, the current thesis aims to characterise associations between brain structural and functional development and individual behavioural variability.

Research into specific neural correlates of literacy and numeracy has proven challenging for several reasons. For instance, any comparison between individuals who perform poorly in either one of these areas with age-matched controls is confounded by schooling. Specifically, typically developing children train the neural systems underlying the respective domains more than impaired individuals. This in itself induces changes in the brain's structural and functional architecture, impeding the direct differentiation between potential causes of disorders and consequences of reduced literacy or numeracy experience (Goswami, 2015; Huettig, Lachmann, Reis, & Petersson, 2018).

When looking at reading, writing and mathematical competence specifically, one of the most significant discussions concerns the question for possible interactions between these abilities. While evidence based on the cognitive profiles of specific impairments suggests two largely independent deficits (Landerl, Fussenegger, Moll, & Willburger, 2009), there is a substantial comorbidity of corresponding learning disorders (Moll, Kunze, Neuhoff, Bruder, & Schulte-Körne, 2014). Moreover, variability in reading and mathematical performance can be partly explained by a common genetic basis (Davis et al., 2014). Thus, when aiming to characterise specific contributions of neural systems to individual differences and deficits in either domain, a careful investigation and rigorous statistical control is necessary to identify effects unique to literacy or numeracy.

The present thesis aims to shed light on networks supporting early literacy and numeracy in the developing brain. To this end, we investigated the brain basis of these complex cognitive abilities in two separate studies using structural and resting-state functional magnetic resonance imaging (MRI). Importantly, the work presented in this thesis relies on longitudinal imaging data obtained from young children, in conjunction with extensive psychometric testing. This design serves as the basis for investigating two distinct key questions: (a) What are neural correlates of deficient literacy acquisition, distinguishing dyslexic children from typically developing controls? (b) Which particular developmental trajectories of cortical surface anatomy are associated with initial numeracy attainment?

Chapter 2 provides an overview of the current literature on literacy and numeracy development, particularly considering theories of DD as an example of a severe neurodevelopmental learning disorder. Further, this chapter will highlight important challenges facing research when studying specific neural correlates of both domains. For instance, performance in literacy and numeracy tasks prominantly covaries (Durand, Hulme, Larkin, & Snowling, 2005; Hart, Petrill, Thompson, & Plomin, 2009; Lundberg & Sterner, 2006; Thompson, Detterman, & Plomin, 1991), such that both domains need to be considered when studying

specific correlates of distinct skills. In addition, possible confounds like sociodemographic status or the quality of individual experience with reading, writing and maths, are often not
accounted for in previous work. Based on these shortcomings,
I formulate the research aims and hypotheses of the empirical
work presented here in Chapter 3. Subsequently, Chapter 4 out-
lines general principles guiding brain maturation, thus providing a theoretical foundation for the developmental processes relevant in the context of longitudinal work in children. We employed MRI to empirically measure brain anatomy and functional coherence in vivo. Therefore, Chapter 5 describes the basic principles of this neuroimaging approach. Additionally, this
chapter gives detailed accounts of the sophisticated imaging processing techniques applied to derive information about specific
neuroanatomical and -functional measures, allowing for a more
comprehensive assessment of neural correlates of complex cognitive abilities. I will report a combined study of structural and
resting-state functional correlates of DD both at a preliterate and
school age in Chapter 6. In contrast, the second empirical study
reported in Chapter 7 focuses on structural developmental trajectories related to individual mathematical abilities. Finally, this
thesis closes with a general discussion on how the present findings add to current models of DD and mathematical learning,
and thus further the understanding of the emergence of complex cognitive abilities in Chapter 8.

CHAPTER 2

LITERACY AND NUMERACY

Humans rely on literacy and numeracy every day. While our modern, technology-driven lifes seem impossible without these skills, one should bear in mind that humans are not naturally born readers or maths experts. In fact, literacy and numeracy are relatively recent cultural inventions: while archaeological discoveries of notch marks on bone artefacts suggest the emergence of primitive counting systems as early as 30,000 BC (D. M. Burton, 2011), first scripts emerged around 3300–3200 BC in the ancient Middle East (Stauder, 2010; Woods, 2010) and the oldest records of mathematical texts date back to 1800–1600 BC (D. M. Burton, 2011). Importantly, both literacy and numeracy are not acquired implicitly[1] in the same way as we learn language, or how to walk. Instead, mastering the abstract symbol systems comprising numerals and letters that represent quantities and spoken language respectively, requires systematic instruction and practice.

---

[1]*Note*: Yet, implicit processes that, for instance, support the automatisation of relevant skills (Rivera, Reiss, Eckert, & Menon, 2005; Schwanenflugel et al., 2006) do play a major role for some aspects of literacy and numeracy acquisition.

Considering the fundamental importance of these competencies for later academic success (Duncan et al., 2007), it is not surprising that behavioural and neurobiological correlates of both typical and atypical literacy and numeracy processing have been studied extensively. Therefore, the aim of the present chapter is to provide an overview of current models describing the emergence of literacy on the one hand and numeracy on the other, including literature elucidating their brain basis. For literacy in particular, theories of developmental dyslexia as an example of a severe neurodevelopmental learning disorder are described in Section 2.1.2.1. While the empirical work presented in this thesis comprises two distinct studies investigating neural correlates of individual variation within the two domains independently from each other, it is important to appreciate potential connections between emerging literacy and numeracy skills. Accordingly, the chapter closes with an account of possible associations between them (see Section 2.3), followed by an illustration of further confounds that pose challenges for research (see Section 2.4).

2.1   FOUNDATIONS OF LITERACY

Literacy learning constitutes a complex process involving diverse cognitive abilities such as basic visual processing, language processing, learning and memory (Vellutino, Fletcher, Snowling, & Scanlon, 2004). To successfully acquire this ability, the beginning reader needs to grasp the so-called alphabetic principle:

written words consist of subunits (i.e. letters) and there are systematic correspondences between these letters and the sounds of
a language. Understanding this principle requires phonological
awareness, i.e. the ability to split spoken words into their respective constituents (i.e. phonemes) and to manipulate them. Profi-
ciency at analysing and modifying the sound structure of spoken language emerges first in preschool children and develops
gradually during childhood (Liberman & Shankweiler, 1985), establishing the basis of successful early letter-sound decoding.

With instruction and practice, the associations between
speech sounds and visual symbols become more complex, such
that individual phonemes get mapped to groups of letters (i.e.
graphemes). Moreover, they include an increasing proportion of
opaque orthographic rules, such as the digraph "ph" that maps
to the sound /f/ in English. Finally, with more advanced reading experience, whole strings of graphemes get stored in memory. Thus, an orthographic lexicon interfacing with the semantic
system is built. As this lexicon grows, the emerging reader increasingly relies on whole word recognition rather than sequen-
tial phonological decoding of individual graphemes.

One of the prominent models depicting the mental mecha-
nisms involved in reading is the dual-route-cascaded model (see
Figure 2.1; Coltheart, Rastle, Perry, Langdon, & Ziegler, 2001)[2].
Words stored in the orthographic lexicon activate either a lexical-

---

[2]*Note*: Examples for other models include connectionist triangle models
(Harm & Seidenberg, 1999; Plaut, McClelland, Seidenberg, & Patterson,
1996; Seidenberg & McClelland, 1989), the connectionist dual process model
(Zorzi, Houghton, & Butterworth, 1998), and upgraded versions thereof
(Perry, Ziegler, & Zorzi, 2007, 2010).

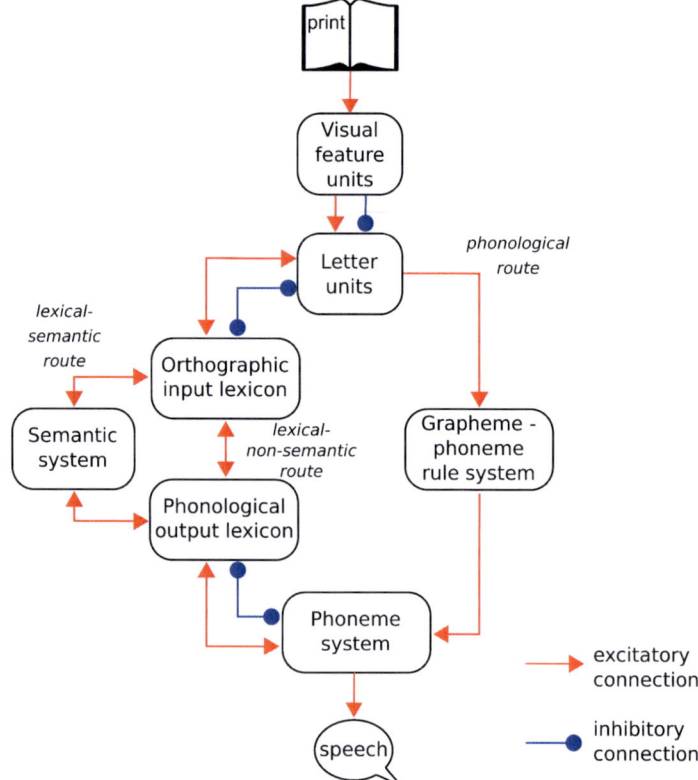

Figure 2.1: The dual-route cascaded model of visual word recognition and reading aloud. Adapted from "DRC: A dual route cascaded model of visual word recognition and reading aloud" by M. Coltheart, K. Rastle, and C. Perry, 2001, *Psychological Review*, *108*, p. 214. Copyright 2001 by the APA. Adapted with permission.

semantic path, accessing its meaning and its pronunciation, or a lexical non-semantic route, generating its mere pronunciation (see left part of Figure 2.1). In contrast, for novel words that are not stored in the lexicon, the system falls back onto decoding via cross-modal integration along the phonological route (see right part of Figure 2.1): each grapheme gets sequentially mapped onto its corresponding phoneme according to the acquired grapheme-phoneme-rule system.

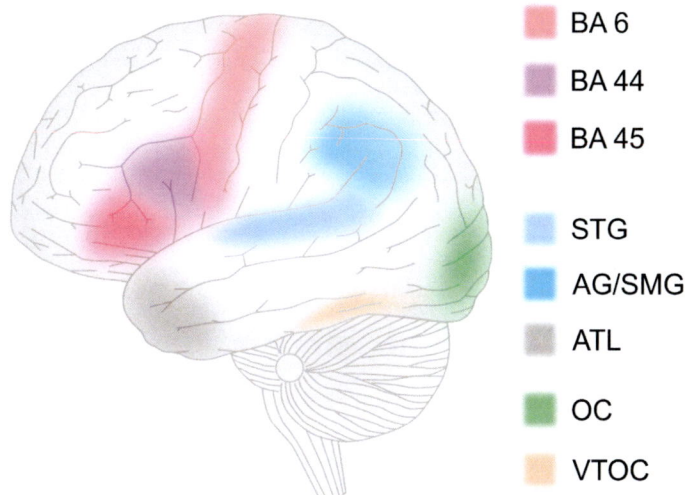

BA 6

BA 44

BA 45

STG

AG/SMG

ATL

OC

VTOC

Figure 2.2: Brain areas associated with reading. Literacy-related networks are typically left-lateralised, thus only the left hemisphere is shown. BA = Brodmann area; STG = superior temporal gyrus; AG/SMG = angular gyrus / supramarginal gyrus; ATL = anterior temporal lobe; OC = occipital cortex; VTOC = ventral temporal-occipital cortex.

2.1.1   *The brain basis of literacy*

The advent of modern, non-invasive neuroimaging tools like MRI permitted researchers to investigate which brain areas are typically involved in reading. This research identified a typically left-lateralised network comprising inferior frontal regions (spanning Brodmann areas 44, 45 and 6), temporoparietal areas such as the angular gyrus, the supramarginal gyrus and the posterior portion of the superior temporal gyrus, and the occipital and ventral temporal-occipital cortex (Pugh et al., 2001, see Figure 2.2). Further evidence suggests a dissociation of this system into a dorsal and a ventral reading network, respectively (Jobard, Crivello, & Tzourio-Mazoyer, 2003; Schlaggar & McCandliss, 2007).

The left ventral temporal-occipital cortex—specifically the print-sensitive visual word form area (VWFA Cohen et al., 2000)—has been associated with pre-lexical processing of written words (Jobard et al., 2003). This notion is supported by evidence for neural representations of orthographic structures within this area (Glezer, Jiang, & Riesenhuber, 2009). The ventral temporal-occipital cortex is connected to temporoparietal and inferior frontal regions via the arcuate fasciculus (de Schotten, Cohen, Amemiya, Braga, & Dehaene, 2014), forming the dorsal reading network. Functionally, the temporal and anterior regions involved in reading are prominently associated with phonological processing. For instance, the posterior part of the inferior frontal gyrus (i.e., BA44) was shown to be active in tasks requiring the analysis of phonological consituents of words (Poldrack et al., 1999). Like the left ventral premotor cortex (i.e., BA6), this region has also been implicated in recoding phonological information into corresponding articulatory motor plans (M. W. Burton, LoCasto, Krebs-Noble, & Gullapalli, 2005; C. J. Price, 2012). Together with posterior BA44, temporoparietal regions like the left supramarginal gyrus and superior temporal areas showed higher activation in phonological compared to semantic decision tasks (McDermott, Petersen, Watson, & Ojemann, 2003) and stronger responses during reading of pseudowords (Borowsky et al., 2006). Furthermore, the posterior superior temporal cortex was shown to exhibit heteromodal responses to both letter and speech sound stimuli, integrating visual and auditory speech information (van Atteveldt, Formisano,

Goebel, & Blomert, 2004). Consequently, the dorsal route is assumed to underly the the integration of orthographic and phonological information (Jobard et al., 2003; Preston et al., 2016).

The ventral route, in contrast, links the temporal-occipital cortex with regions involved in semantic processing (Carreiras, Armstrong, Perea, & Frost, 2014). Specifically, this route projects along the anterior temporal lobe and the ventral part of the inferior frontal gyrus (i.e. BA45) via the inferior fronto-occipital fasciculus. The anterior temporal lobe has been characterised as an amodal semantic system, with overlapping activity for pictures, speech and print (Visser, Jefferies, & Lambon Ralph, 2010). Similarly, the ventral inferior frontal gyrus showed preferential activation during semantic processing compared to phonological processing (Poldrack et al., 1999). Consequently, this ventral route has been associated with the integration of orthographic and semantic information.[3]

2.1.2 *Developmental dyslexia*

Developmental dyslexia (DD), a severe deficit in literacy acquisition, is one of the most common specific learning disorders listed in the International Classification of Diseases (World Health Organization, 2018) with reported prevalence rates ranging from 3–17% of the population (Barbiero et al., 2012; S. E. Shaywitz et al., 1998). The first scientific accounts of this deficit date back

---

[3]*Note*: Integration of semantic and orthographic information is not restricted to this ventral route, as semantic processing during reading also engages the angular gyrus (C. J. Price & Mechelli, 2005), indicating a corresponding role for a further dorsal connection.

over 140 years ago. After initial reports of "word-blindness" by German physician Adolf Kußmaul in 1877 (Kußmaul, 1877), his compatriot, ophthalmologist Rudolf Berlin, coined the term "Dyslexia" as a severe impairment of reading abilities in 1887 (Berlin, 1887). Nearly a decade later, the British physician W. Pringle Morgan described the case of a 14-year old boy of average intelligence and vision, who nevertheless struggled severely with reading and spelling (Morgan, 1896). Remarkably, this boy did not have a history of brain lesions or head trauma. As a specific developmental learning disorder, the pathology of DD must neither be attributable to intellectual disability, inadequate instruction or schooling, or sensory impairment regarding vision or hearing (S. E. Shaywitz, 1998; Vellutino et al., 2004; World Health Organization, 2018).

2.1.2.1   *Cognitive deficits and neurobiological theories*

Persistent impairments in literacy learning—affecting reading, spelling or both—are at the core of DD. Specifically, reading difficulties are expressed in terms of significantly decreased reading speed, accuracy and comprehension, while spelling deficits comprise frequent capitalization errors, elisions or substitutions of graphemes (Schulte-Körne, 2010).

Interestingly, many individuals with dyslexia show co-occurring problems in terms of phonological, low-level sensory, and motor processing. Based on these variable cognitive profiles exhibited by dyslexic individuals, multiple attempts have been made to explain DD, while also accounting for the concurrent deficits. A number of these accounts make specific predictions about the neurobiological underpinnings of DD: (i) the phonological deficit theory, (ii) the cerebellar deficit theory, (iii) sensory processing deficit theories, and (iv) the magnocellular deficit theory. The remainder of this section provides an overview of cognitive impairments prominently observed in dyslexic individuals in the context of the above-mentioned theories. Furthermore, supporting as well as conflicting evidence from neuroanatomical, electrophysiological and neuroimaging studies is presented.

THE PHONOLOGICAL DEFICIT THEORY.   Individuals suffering from DD show persistently poor performance in tasks requiring phonological awareness, phonological short-term and working memory (Snowling, 1998). These tasks include rhyming, phoneme deletion, non-word repetition, or rapid automatised naming (Landerl et al., 2009; Lehongre, Ramus, Villiermet, Schwartz, & Giraud, 2011; Ramus et al., 2003; Snowling, Muter, & Carroll, 2007).

Importantly, adequate phonological awareness skills are necessary to be able to reliably separate a spoken word into its phonologic constituents represented as alphabetic characters in script (S. E. Shaywitz et al., 1998). Consequently, the phonological deficit theory posits that poor phonological skills inhibit the development of reliable phoneme-grapheme mapping abilities. Thus, beginning readers struggle to build the associations between letters and their corresponding sounds, which in turn im-

pedes syllable and ultimately whole-word recognition, hinder-
ing fluent literacy acquisition (Snowling, 1998).

Among the accounts arguing for a unique causal factor in
the emergence of DD, the phonological deficit theory has received the most attention (Vellutino et al., 2004) and gains support from various studies identifying structural and functional
anomalies in the dorsal reading network of dyslexic individuals. In early post mortem histological work, Galaburda, Sherman, Rosen, Aboitiz, and Geschwind (1985) identified small ac-
cumulations of neurons—so-called ectopias—generally in perisylvian cortical areas. Predominantly, these were located in the
typically cell-free layer I of the respective regions. Moreover, the
dyslexic individuals exhibited polymicrogyria, i. e. a disproportionate number of small cortical foldings, within the planum
temporale and posterior superior temporal gyrus. Finally, the investigated brains were marked by deviant patterns of symmetrical plana temporale instead of the commonly observed left-ward
asymmetry. In line with this post mortem examination, a meta-
analysis of structural neuroimaging studies identified dyslexia-
specific reductions in grey matter volume of the posterior superior temporal sulcus (Richlan, Kronbichler, & Wimmer, 2013).
Moreover, deficits in phonological awareness have been linked
to the structure of the arcuate fasciculus, the dorsal white matter connection supporting phonological processing (Saygin et al.,
2013; Vandermosten et al., 2012). In addition, DD has been functionally associated with hypoactivation of the dorsal reading net-

work during phonological processing (Paulesu et al., 1996; Pugh et al., 2000; Richlan, Kronbichler, & Wimmer, 2009).

While many agree that a phonological deficit plays a key role in the emergence of DD, its exact nature remains elusive. For instance, Boets et al. (2013) demonstrated robust and distinct phonological representations in adults with dyslexia. Instead, these authors suggested an impairment of access of otherwise intact representations, based on the observation of hampered functional and structural connectivity between the left inferior frontal and temporoparietal cortex. In contrast, another line of research suggests impaired phonological representations based on variable neural responses to speech sounds within the primary auditory cortex (Lehongre et al., 2011).

Despite the widely recognised contribution of phonological deficits to reading impairment, their role as the sole cause of DD has been questioned. One line of criticism drew attention to dyslexic cases without a phonological disorder (Bosse, Tainturier, & Valdois, 2007; Peyrin et al., 2012) and the fact that not all individuals with literacy difficulties depict equally strong phonological problems (R. L. Peterson, Pennington, Olson, & Wadsworth, 2014). Moreover, the phonological deficit theory has also been criticised for failing to account for co-occurring sensory (Lovegrove, Bowling, Badcock, & Blackwood, 1980) and motor deficits (Nicolson & Fawcett, 1990) observed in dyslexic individuals.

THE CEREBELLAR DEFICIT THEORY.   In addition to com-
promised phonological processing, some studies reported impairments in the maintenance of posture and balance (Fawcett
& Nicolson, 1999; Fawcett, Nicolson, & Dean, 1996; Nicolson
& Fawcett, 1994) and implicit sequence learning (Howard Jr.,
Howard, Japikse, & Eden, 2005; Stoodley, Ray, Jack, & Stein,
2008; Vicari, Marotta, Menghini, Molinari, & Petrosini, 2003)
in some dyslexic individuals. These observations lend support
to the cerebellar deficit theory, suggesting that dyslexia-specific
problems follow from a more general inability to fully automa-
tise skills (Nicolson & Fawcett, 1990). Specifically, this account
suggests that impairments of the cerebellum and the cerebro-
cerebellar loop cause deficits in motor, articulatory and automatisation skills, in turn impeding writing, reading and spelling
abilities (Nicolson & Fawcett, 2005; Nicolson, Fawcett, & Dean,
2001). Consequently, poor phonological abilities prominently associated with dyslexia are assumed to follow from a more fundamental cerebellar deficit.

In support of this theory, Finch, Nicolson, and Fawcett (2002)
reported atypical cell distributions in the anterior and posterior
cerebellar lobes of four dyslexic males investigated post mortem.
Further neuroimaging evidence suggested reduced grey matter
volume of the cerebellum in dyslexic individuals (Eckert et al.,
2003; Eckert et al., 2005). Moreover, Nicolson et al. (1999) and
Nicolson et al. (2001) proposed a cerebellar dysfunction as a
potential functional substrate for dyslexia, based on evidence

of significantly reduced activation in dyslexic adults when performing a motor-sequence learning task.

However, the cerebellar deficit hypothesis has been met with scepticism, mainly due to the inconsistency of findings. For instance, S. White et al. (2006), comparing groups of dyslexic, autistic, and control children that were matched for age and nonverbal IQ, found motor impairments in some, but not all, dyslexic children. Moreover, a subgroup of the autistic children also displayed deficits in the execution of tasks tapping into manual dexterity and balance skills, but lacked reading impairments. Similarly, Savage et al. (2005) demonstrated that performance on a postural stability task did not reliably discriminate between poor, average, and good readers. Finally, in a recent study, van Oers et al. (2018) compared adult dyslexics with controls in an attempt to investigate the cerebellar involvement in dyslexia. While dyslexics did indeed show worse performance on tasks requiring sound cerebellar function, there was no relationship between behavioural deficits and grey matter volume of this brain region. Against this background, these authors oppose the notion of a causal involvement of a cerebellum in DD.

SENSORY PROCESSING THEORIES.   While acknowledging the dominant role of phonological deficits in DD, a number of authors put forward the idea that these problems are secondary to more basic disturbances of visual or auditory systems.

In one of the first accounts of dyslexia, Kußmaul (1877) cued the term "word-blindness" for severe and unexpected reading

impairment. Indeed, literacy critically depends on reliable identification of visually presented symbols. In addition, differences
between skilled readers and dyslexic individuals in terms of
basic visual processing have been reported. For instance, Lovegrove et al. (1980) demonstrated diminished contrast sensitivity in reading impaired participants compared to controls, suggesting disruptions in the cortical circuits associated with primary visual function in DD. Further, dyslexic individuals were
shown to experience greater interference from surrounding elements when looking at arrays of symbols, so-called 'visual
crowding' effects, and to benefit from increased inter-letter spac-
ing (Spinelli, De Luca, Judica, & Zoccolotti, 2002). Bosse et al.
(2007), based on a study of French and British children, suggested that a reduced visual attention span limits the amount of
information that can be sustained, thus hampering reading acquisition independently from phonological deficits. Others characterised the nature of a visual impairment in terms of deficient
visuospatial attention control (Facoetti et al., 2003; Facoetti et al.,
2006), positing that dyslexic individuals fail to shift their focus
of attention smoothly across printed text.

Several studies provide evidence for neural correlates of visual deficits in dyslexia. In an electroencephalography (EEG) experiment, adult dyslexics showed reduced responses to rapid,
low-contrast stimulation (Livingstone, Rosen, Drislane, & Galaburda, 1991). Importantly, Livingstone et al. complemented
these findings with a post mortem examination of the lateral
geniculate nucleus (LGN), a subpart of the thalamus respon-

sible for visual processing. Specifically, dyslexic autopsy specimens exhibited disorganised magnocellular layers and reduced
cell size within this thalamic nucleus. Moreover, evidence from
functional magnetic resonance imaging (fMRI) suggested diminished visual motion sensitivity within the middle temporal area
of adult dyslexic individuals (Eden et al., 1996). Further, Peyrin
et al. (2012) presented the case of a dyslexic individual with an
impaired visual attention span but preserved phonological skills,
demonstrating hypoactivation of parietal lobules during a visual
categorization task. Taken together, these studies support the notion of an underlying visual deficit in DD.

A different line of argumentation characterised deficits in basic auditory perception as an underlying cause of poor phonological skills. Based on behavioural evidence suggesting a relation between literacy problems and impaired processing of brief
or rapidly changing acoustic stimulation (Helenius, Uutela, &
Hari, 1999; Tallal, 1980), the auditory deficit theory posits that
dyslexic individuals fail to detect subtle differences in the sound
stream like the distinction between 'bath' and 'path'. In addition,
several studies demonstrated poor performance of dyslexic individuals with respect to processing prosody-related (Foxton et
al., 2003; Goswami et al., 2002; Richardson, Thomson, Scott, &
Goswami, 2004) and more general acoustic features (Baldeweg,
Richardson, Watkins, Foale, & Gruzelier, 1999).

The notion of a fundamental auditory deficit was supported
by Galaburda, Menard, and Rosen (1994), identifying atypical
right-left asymmetry of the medial geniculate body (MGB), i.e.

the auditory sensory thalamus: the left MGB contained significantly more smaller neurons compared to typical samples in five dyslexic autopsy specimens. Corroborating this initial structural finding, Díaz, Hintz, Kiebel, and von Kriegstein (2012) reported a dysfunction of the MGB when participants were asked to attend to speech sound changes, suggesting a neurobiological correlate of rapid sensory processing deficits in DD. In line with this, Hornickel and Kraus (2013) demonstrated unstable neural responses to sound within the inferior colliculus of the brainstem.

Nevertheless, the overall causal role of sensory deficits for DD has been criticised (Vellutino et al., 2004). For instance, a number of studies failed to replicate auditory (Halliday & Bishop, 2006; Hämäläinen et al., 2009; Hill, Bailey, Griffiths, & Snowling, 1999; Kronbichler, Hutzler, & Wimmer, 2002) or visual (Johannes, Kussmaul, Münte, & Mangun, 1996; Kronbichler et al., 2002; Williams, Stuart, Castles, & McAnally, 2003) deficits in dyslexic individuals, or detected these only for a subgroup of the investigated samples (Amitay, Ben-Yehudah, Banai, & Ahissar, 2002; Bosse et al., 2007; Rosen & Manganari, 2001; Tallal, 1980; S. White et al., 2006).

Particularly compelling evidence for a causal association between sensory deficits and dyslexia comes from accounts of structural abnormality of thalamic nuclei mentioned above (Galaburda et al., 1994; Livingstone et al., 1991). Remarkably, however, there is experimental evidence for the occurence of such sub-cortical structural anomalies as a consequence of cortical malformation. Herman, Galaburda, Fitch, Carter, and Rosen (1997), inducing small lesions in bilateral prefrontal, parietal or occipital cortices of new–born rats, demonstrated that these anomalies led to changes in cell size distribution of the MGB in male, but not female, animals. Importantly, these changes resembled the aberrant neuronal distribution observed in human dyslexic autopsy specimen (Galaburda et al., 1994). Moreover, the lesioned male rats were also significantly impaired in their ability to perform fast auditory discrimination.

Overall, despite criticism and evidence to the contrary, sensory deficits remain viable and prominent candidates potentially contributing to the development of literacy impairments.

THE MAGNOCELLULAR DEFICIT THEORY.   In an attempt to integrate the variable findings concerning impairments in the visual, auditory and motor domain, Stein and Walsh (1997) formulated the magnocellular deficit theory as an overarching account.

The magnocellular theory was first defined based on the distinction of the visual system into magnocellular and parvocellular branches, processing rapid, low-contrast and slow, high-contrast sensory information, respectively (Livingstone & Hubel, 1988). Structural abnormalities of the visual thalamus (i.e., the LGN) in dyslexic individuals reported by Livingstone et al. (1991) were in fact restricted to magnocellular layers. Integrating these findings with evidence of reduced visual contrast sensitivity (Hoeft et al., 2007), hypoactivation of motion-sensitive cortical regions (Eden et al., 1996), auditory temporal dysfunction (Helenius et al., 1999; Tallal, 1980) and poor performance in cerebellar tasks (Nicolson & Fawcett, 1994), the magnocellular theory suggests a fundamental, cross-modal core deficit in temporal processing in DD (Stein, 2001, 2018; Stein & Talcott, 1999; Stein & Walsh, 1997). Following this account, the detrimental impact of low-level anomalies extends to more high-level domains, for instance also affecting visuospatial attention in the posterior parietal cortex (PPC; Stein, 2001). Therefore, impaired temporal processing along magnocellular pathways within different modalities was hypothesised to affect not merely one, but multiple domains, thereby explaining the variable profiles of DD.

However, this theory faces criticism comparable to the proposals presented above, failing to account for any study that does not find visual, auditory or cerebellar magnocellular deficits in dyslexic individuals. Additionally, it struggles to explain more general perceptual impairments going beyond the magnocellular system (Amitay et al., 2002). Furthermore, Sabine Heim, Freeman Jr., Eulitz, and Elbert (2001) presented evidence suggesting that in some dyslexic individuals, sensory deficits do not extend across multiple domains, opposing the notion of a general cross-modal temporal processing impairment. Thus, the claim for a causal role of magnocellular deficits as the cause of DD remains contentious.

2.1.2.2 *Disentangling potential causes from consequences of developmental dyslexia*

The diverse list of theories described in Section 2.1.2.1 elucidates that much debate and little agreement exists regarding the causal neurobiological deficits of DD. Based on results from data driven clustering approaches, some authors argued for a division into subgroups derived from distinctive cognitive profiles in order to account for its multifactorial nature (Stefan Heim et al., 2008; King, Giess, & Lombardino, 2007; Morris et al., 1998). While such behavioural subdivisions have significant implications for educational practise and remediation, the question whether distinct cognitive profiles can be traced back to distinct neurobiological causes or rather to a sole root dysfunction remains unanswered.

Successfully learning how to read and write is a highly dynamic process, taxing diverse cognitive abilities and inducing widespread changes in the structural (Carreiras et al., 2009; Yeatman, Dougherty, Ben-Shachar, & Wandell, 2012) and functional (Brem et al., 2010; Carreiras et al., 2009; Dehaene et al., 2010; Skeide et al., 2017) architecture of the emerging reader's brain. However, individuals who fall behind in this process will vary in amount and quality of neuroplastic change occuring. Therefore, empirical evidence of neurobiological differences based on school-aged children and adults may confound potential causes of being dyslexic with consequences of reduced reading experience (Goswami, 2015), as individuals with specific learning disorders like DD actively avoid reading-related material (Haft,

Duong, Ho, Hendren, & Hoeft, 2018). This line of argumentation has been recently adopted by Huettig et al. (2018), paralleling cognitive deficits in dyslexic individuals to those observed in illiterates who have no practice in reading.

Study designs comparing affected individuals with age-matched and reading-level matched controls aim to distinguish effects driven by different amount and quality of literacy experience from anomalies related to DD per se (Goswami, 2015). For instance, Hoeft et al. (2007) demonstrated that activation patterns in left inferior and middle frontal gyri, the caudate nucleus, and the thalamus in dyslexic adolescents resemble those exhibited by younger individuals matched in reading performance during a visual rhyme judgment task. Compared to age-matched controls, however, activation in these regions was significantly higher, reflecting differences in current literacy ability unrelated to the aetiology of DD. Instead, reduced activity in left fusiform and parietal areas and smaller grey matter volume in a region of interest in left inferior parietal cortex distinguished dyslexics from both control groups. In a whole-brain analysis, Krafnick, Flowers, Luetje, Napoliello, and Eden (2014) reported reduced cortical volume of the right precentral cortex and increased grey matter volume of the left middle temporal gyrus in dyslexic children compared to younger controls with comparable reading levels. Recently, A. J. Power, Colling, Mead, Barnes, and Goswami (2016) demonstrated poor encoding of speech sounds in literacy impaired children compared to age- and reading-level matched controls. This is in line with previous accounts of variable neural responses to speech sounds within the primary auditory cortex of dyslexic adults (Lehongre et al., 2011). Taken together, these findings might point to a fundamental role of inaccurate neuronal representation of prosodic and syllabic information at level of the primary auditory and superior temporal cortex.

However, evidence provided by reading-level matched designs—despite being a valuable tool—requires cautious interpretation. Improved metacognitive skills in older children might mask behavioural differences actually present between dyslexic individuals and younger controls (Goswami, 2015). Moreover, behavioural measures might be not equally reliable, discriminative and valid across different age groups, raising doubt about the validity of comparisons (Jackson & Butterfield, 1989).

The gold-standard solution for establishing causality is to employ longitudinal designs continuously monitoring behaviour and brain development of children from an early, pre-reading age until after the onset of literacy instruction (Goswami, 2015; Ramus, Altarelli, Jednoróg, Zhao, & Scotto di Covella, 2018). Thus, based on the knowledge of future individual learning progression, neural precursors of DD can be identified from data acquired at a pre-reading age. Due to their effortful nature, however, such designs are sparse. A seminal MRI study by Clark et al. (2014) investigated changes in cortical thickness in children with dyslexia and controls from pre-school age until grade six in school. Their results suggested that children later developing dyslexia have a significantly thinner cortical ribbon in left Heschl's gyrus, lingual gyrus, medial frontal gyrus, middle cingulate gyrus and right orbitofrontal cortex already before formal reading instruction. Moreover, cortical thickness in dyslexic individuals remained significantly smaller in Heschl's and lingual gyrus throughout development, while differences in frontal and cingulate regions disappeared over time. Thus, Clark et al. (2014) suggest a key role of neuroanatomical anomalies in lower-level areas responsible for auditory and visual processing for the aetiology of DD. However, this account has been criticised because of low statistical power and lack of control for genetic factors and environmental variance such as parental education (Kraft et al., 2015). Furthermore, children were 6-7 years old and already attending grade 1 of school at the time of the first scanning, raising doubts whether the presented data can disentangle potential causes from consequence entirely (Ramus et al., 2018).

In summary, potential neural causes and consequences of DD have been the subject of intense debate within the scientific community. To date, there is no general agreement which of the proposed theories captures the fundamental causes of literacy impairments. The most prominent shortcoming in this debate concerns the fact that data supporting or opposing the different accounts is derived from individuals past the age of reading acquisition. What is more, the sparse neuroimaging data available (Clark et al., 2014) is limited to a neo-cortical thickness analysis, thus failing to provide insights into variable neuroanatomical and -functional profiles potentially extending to subcortical systems. Therefore, the work presented in this thesis was designed to overcome these limitations. Specifically, the first empirical study presented here (see Chapter 6) relies on a longitudinal data set comprising various brain structural and functional measures and psychometric testing of the same dyslexic and typically reading children at kindergarten and school age.

2.2   FOUNDATIONS OF NUMERACY

Already early in life, prelinguistic infants as young as six months of age exhibit the ability to differentiate between sets of different magnitudes (F. Xu & Spelke, 2000). Thus, a sense for number is available in early childhood, preceding any formal instruction of numerical concepts (Dehaene, 2011).

One crucial mechanism assumed to support such an innate number sense is the mental number line in the brain. This concept assumes that—independent of modality (Lipton & Spelke, 2003)—magnitudes are coded spatially. Following this account, differences between two sets are represented as the spatial interval separating the two given quantities (Dehaene, 2011; Moyer & Landauer, 1967; Slaughter, Kamppi, & Paynter, 2006). Thereby, the mental number line provides a cross-modal basis for approximate number estimation (Feigenson, Dehaene, & Spelke, 2004). Early support for an intrinsic association between coding of space and magnitude was provided by Dehaene, Bossini, and Giraux (1993), who demonstrated a marked left-ward advantage in terms of reaction time for responding to smaller quantities, and a right-ward advantage for larger values.

A second fundamental mechanism concerns accurate representation of a limited number of items early in life (Feigenson et al., 2004). For instance, Feigenson, Carey, and Hauser (2002) demonstrated that ten- and 12-month-old infants instinctively select the larger set when making one versus two or two versus three comparisons. This finding suggests infants' ability to track a small number of discrete objects correctly (Bremner et al., 2017; Feigenson et al., 2002).

Over development, these two mechanisms mature, increasing in precision (Lipton & Spelke, 2003) and eventually enabling preschoolers to perform approximate addition (Barth et al., 2006; Barth et al., 2005) and subtraction (Slaughter et al., 2006). However, development of skills needed for exact symbolic arithmetic requires formal instruction in school (Barth et al., 2005). Importantly, these developmental trajectories are characterised by marked inter-individual variability in learning rates and success (M. Brown et al., 2003; Cockcroft, 1982).

Finally, there is a consensus that—during development of numerical and mathematical competence in school—children shift from procedural approaches such as counting to memory-based retrieval strategies to solve simple mathematical equations (Ashcraft, 1982; Barrouillet & Fayol, 1998; Siegler & Shipley, 1995). Specifically, Qin et al. (2014), investigating arithmetic problem solving strategies in children, adolescents and adults, showed that this shift gradually progresses during childhood and further through adolescence into adulthood.

2.2.1 *The brain basis of numeracy*

The ability to engage with and manipulate quantitative information rests upon biologically determined circuits for magnitude and number processing (Dehaene, Piazza, Pinel, & Cohen, 2003). However, much like literacy, numerical cognition taps into multiple cognitive domains. Beyond core magnitude and number processing, it involves working memory, vision, cognitive control, attention and memory (Menon, 2015). Consequently, a diverse range of brain regions has been associated with its development, such as the prefrontal cortex (PFC; Cho, Ryali, Geary, & Menon, 2011; Evans et al., 2015; Rivera et al., 2005), the posterior parietal cortex (PPC; Cantlon, Brannon, Carter, & Pelphrey, 2006; Menon, 2010; Qin et al., 2014; Rivera et al., 2005) including the intraparietal sulcus (IPS; Cantlon et al., 2006; Jolles, Ashkenazi, et al., 2016), the medial temporal lobe (MTL; Cho et al., 2011; Qin et al., 2014; Rivera et al., 2005; Supekar et al., 2013), and the ventral temporal-occipital cortex (VTOC; Evans et al., 2015; Rivera et al., 2005).

Importantly, previous developmental studies shed light onto structural and functional changes within these areas while mathematical competence matures. In a cross-sectional analysis, Rivera et al. (2005) investigated neural correlates of developmental changes in mental arithmetic during late childhood and adolescence. Their results suggested a consistent decrease of prefrontal activation, reflecting reduced reliance on effortful strategies tapping into working memory and attentional re-

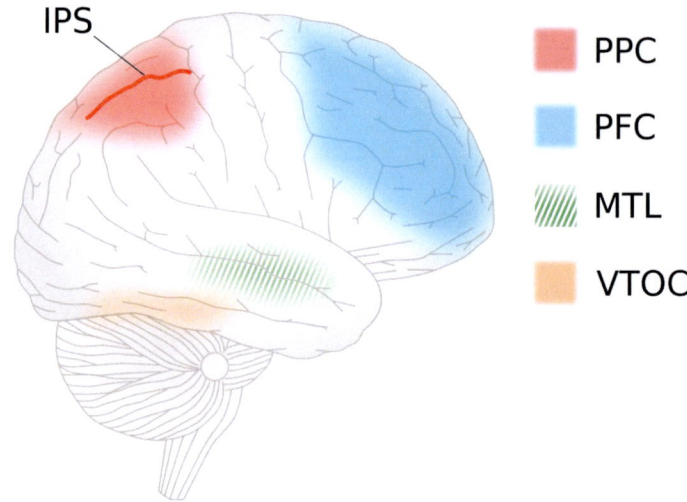

Figure 2.3: Brain areas associated with numeracy processing. PPC = posterior parietal cortex; PFC = prefrontal cortex; MTL = medial temporal lobe; VTOC = ventral temporal-occipital cortex, IPS = intraparietal sulcus. Regions are schematically shown for the right hemisphere, but importance of bilateral areas is prominently reported.

sources. Concomitantly, involvement of regions specialised for mathematical processing, such as the left supramarginal gyrus and anterior IPS, increased with time and experience. This finding was corroborated by Evans et al. (2015), who showed that the longitudinal change in parietal grey matter volume, together with ventral temporal and prefrontal areas, predicted improvement of mathematical abilities in children between seven and 14 years of age. Moreover, PPC regions are consistently associated with magnitude processing (Piazza, Izard, Pinel, Le Bihan, & Dehaene, 2004; Piazza, Mechelli, Price, & Butterworth, 2006; Piazza, Pinel, Le Bihan, & Dehaene, 2007) and mental arithmetic (Knops, Thirion, Hubbard, Michel, & Dehaene, 2009; Menon, 2010; Venkatraman, Ansari, & Chee, 2005) in adults, even in absence of an explicit task (Ansari, Dhital, & Siong, 2006). Specifically, Dehaene et al. (2003) distinguished three distinct modules in the parietal cortex crucial for sound numerical cognition. Following this account, the horizontal segment of the IPS represents a domain specific core quantity region that can be considered to house the neural representation of the mental number line mentioned in Section 2.2. Importantly, developmental work indicates differential hemispheric trajectories: While four-year-old children already exhibit adult-like levels of activation in right IPS (Cantlon et al., 2006), its left homologue increases in functional specialisation with age (Rivera et al., 2005). In line with this previous finding, Jolles, Supekar, et al. (2016) associated increased functional connectivity of the left IPS with individual improvement when solving simple addition and subtraction problems in primary school children after an 8-week intense math tutoring program. Second, bilateral posterior superior parietal regions seem to play a more domain general role. While these regions are differentially activated during counting (Piazza, Mechelli, Butterworth, & Price, 2002) and mathematical operations (Rosenberg-Lee, Chang, Young, Wu, & Menon, 2011), they are also prominently associated with visuospatial processing, attention and short-term memory (Corbetta, Kincade, Ollinger, McAvoy, & Shulman, 2000; Ester, Sprague, & Serences, 2015; Simon, Mangin, Cohen, Le Bihan, & Dehaene, 2002). Therefore, Dehaene et al. described the bilateral superior parietal cortex as an auxiliary system, providing attentional orientation along the mental number line. Finally, as part of the left-hemispheric perisylvian system, the left angular gyrus has been shown to be involved in phoneme detection tasks as well as calculation (Simon et al., 2002). Moreover, it activates more strongly in simple one-digit multiplication tasks that can be solved via retrieval of arithmetic facts compared to multi-digit multiplication requiring quantity manipulation (Grabner et al., 2007). This finding is in line with the suggested involvement of the angular gyrus in verbal manipulation of number and arithmetic fact retrieval (Dehaene et al., 2003).

MTL involvement follows a non-linear trajectory. Hippocampal activation initially increases when children first develop memory-based retrieval strategies, followed by a reduction during adolescence reflecting final consolidation (Qin et al., 2014). This is in line with evidence indicating that larger hippocampal volume predicts learning improvements after intensive math tutoring (Supekar et al., 2013). Moreover, variable neural representations in MTL distinguished children that rely more on fact retrieval from those who employ procedural strategies (e. g. counting; Cho et al., 2011).

Lastly, ventral temporal-occipital cortex (VTOC) regions have been recently associated with symbolic numerical cognition in terms of a visual number form area that specifically decodes visual numerals (Amalric & Dehaene, 2016; Hermes et al., 2017; Shum et al., 2013). However, the concept of a region specifically tuned to digits is under debate. For instance, G. R. Price and Ansari (2011) failed to observe any digit-specific activation in VTOC and instead ascribe a numeral-specific role to the angular gyrus. While such a null result might be due to signal drop out specifically affecting ventral areas (Yeo, Wilkey, & Price, 2017), there is yet little agreement about the exact localisation or role of this region. Based on a meta-analysis of neuroimaging studies, Yeo et al. (2017) identified common numeral-specific tuning of the right inferior temporal gyrus in addition to a network of areas involved in symbolic number processing. Even though this finding aligns with results of Grotheer, Ambrus, and Kovács (2016), demonstrating that transcranial magnetic stimulation of the right—but not left—number form region disrupts visual perception of Arabic numerals, it is noteworthy that stimulation also interfered with letter processing. In fact, Grotheer, Jeska, and Grill-Spector (2018), investigating the functional specificity of candidate VTOC regions, recently reported tuning to numerical content of visual stimuli rather than numerals per se. Thus, while VTOC activation is consistently reported across studies, its exact role for numerical cognition remains contentious.

In summary, the brain basis of numerical-mathematical processing has been intensely studied in adult participants (Ansari et al., 2006; Knops et al., 2009; Menon, 2010; Piazza et al., 2004; Piazza et al., 2006; Piazza et al., 2007; Qin et al., 2014; Venkatraman et al., 2005). From a neurodevelopmental perspective, specific correlates of basic numerical processing and mathematical learning have been investigated in independent samples of preschoolers (Cantlon et al., 2006) and primary school children (Evans et al., 2015; Qin et al., 2014; Rivera et al., 2005), respectively. However, little is known about the longitudinal neuroplastic changes that underlie emerging mathematical skills at the transition from kindergarten to the first years of school. Therefore, the second study presented in this thesis (see Chapter 7) longitudinally assessed the association between cortical surface changes from kindergarten to school age and individual differences in numeracy attainment.

2.3   POTENTIAL LINKS BETWEEN LITERACY AND NUMERACY

At first sight, the ability to read and write seems to be very different from the capacity to apply and reason with numerical concepts. However, both sound literacy and numeracy skills are vital, as letters and numbers belong to the primary means of communication in our modern world. What is more, when considering the two domains, several common features become apparent. Ultimately, both are—to a great extend—explicitly learned abilities to derive new meaning from incoming sensory input. To do so, both require integration of this novel, symbol-based information with prior knowledge given a particular context. Moreover, both require monitoring of ongoing processes (L. Sammons, 2011). Considering these striking commonalities, a central question concerns possible interactions of both domains.

In fact, significant correlations between literacy and numeracy scores are prominently observed (Durand et al., 2005; Hart et al., 2009; Lundberg & Sterner, 2006; Thompson et al., 1991). For instance, Hecht, Torgesen, Wagner, and Rashotte (2001), examining cognitive abilities of 201 children longitudinally over the first years of school, reported positive associations between scores of reading and simple arithmetic assessed both in fourth and fifth grade. Moreover, school-entry numeracy skills were shown to predict later achievement not just in maths, but also in reading (Duncan et al., 2007). In addition to the association between typical reading and mathematical acquisition, there is also evidence for a possible link regarding the impaired development of these skills. Atypically developing individuals often exhibit combined learning deficits. Owing to variable cut-off criteria and distinct operationalisations of deficits, reported comorbidity rates of literacy and numeracy impairments range from 20% to over 80% (Badian, 1999; Dirks, Spyer, van Lieshout, & de Sonneville, 2008; Fletcher & Loveland, 1986; Lewis, Hitch, & Walker, 1994; Moll, Kunze, et al., 2014; von Aster, Schweiter, & Weinhold Zulauf, 2007). Associations between the two deficits are frequently explained in terms of more general processes involved in both, such as complex language (Purpura, Logan, Hassinger-Das, & Napoli, 2017) and phonological processing skills (De Smedt, Taylor, Archibald, & Ansari, 2010; Hecht et al., 2001), executive functioning underlying cognitive flexibility (Yeniad, Malda, Mesman, van Ijzendoorn, & Pieper, 2013), motivation and focused attention (Lundberg & Sterner, 2006) and visual associative learning (Skeide, Evans, Mei, Abrams, & Menon, 2018).

Studies investigating the heritability of literacy and numeracy abilities suggest a substantial genetic influence contributing to individual performance within each domain (Grasby, Coventry, Byrne, Olson, & Medland, 2016; Kovas, Haworth, Dale, & Plomin, 2007). Large-scale twin studies implied that—not just the variability within—but also the considerable covariation between these areas can be in part explained by a common genetic basis (Davis et al., 2014; Haworth et al., 2009; Wadsworth, De-Fries, Fulker, & Plomin, 1995). In the same vein, hereditary factors explain a significant proportion of covarying literacy and numeracy deficits (Hart et al., 2009; Kovas, Haworth, Harlaar, et al., 2007; Markowitz, Willemsen, Trumbetta, & Boomsma, 2005; Thompson et al., 1991). Specifically, a number of authors supported the notion of a generalist genes hypothesis proposed by Plomin and Kovas (2005), suggesting the same genetic factors affect both typical and atypical performance across domains (Haworth et al., 2009; Kovas, Haworth, Dale, & Plomin, 2007; Kovas, Haworth, Harlaar, et al., 2007).

Few studies are available that contrast neural correlates of isolated and shared disorders. Despite the evidence for considerable comorbidity and shared genetic components, Landerl et al. (2009) argue that both disorders are characterised by distinct deficits. In their study, Landerl et al. compared children with isolated dyslexia and dyscalculia, respectively, to individuals with comorbid impairments and demonstrated a double dissociation: deficits were specific for the distinct subgroups, independent of problems in the respective other domain. Thus, they concluded that underlying problems are domain-specific and not attributable to the same basis. In contrast to this suggestion, however, Skeide et al. (2018) recently identified distinct patterns of cortical folding and functional connectivity of the right parahippocampal gyrus as a common neural substrate of combined deficits.

Overall, research investigating the common basis of both literacy and numeracy in terms of behavioural covariation, genetic factors and neural correlates of isolated and shared disorders has granted valuable insights into possible associations between both domains. The focus of the current dissertation, however, was to study specific neural correlates of individual variation within the two domains independently from performance in the respective other domain. To this end—given the potential links between these two complex cognitive abilities—information of both early literacy and numeracy performance was obtained for all participants under investigation in the present empirical work. This rigorous psychometric assessment enabled the inclusion of measures of early numeracy skills as covariates of no interest when examining potential neural causes of literacy impairments in Empirical Study I (see Chapter 6). Likewise, measures of early reading and spelling performance were included in the analyses of developmental trajectories associated with early mathematical achievement presented in Empirical Study II (see Chapter 7). Thereby, the contributions of specific neural circuits supporting either emerging literacy or numeracy skills were investigated.

2.4   STUDYING LITERACY AND NUMERACY: PROMINENT CONFOUNDS

Aside from the considerable covariance of individual literacy and numeracy abilities described in Section 2.3, performance in both domains may be further affected by a range of other factors. First, academic achievement is related to parental education as an indicator of sociodemographic status, with the mother's highest qualification most strongly impacting cognitive outcomes especially in young children (Carneiro, Meghir, & Parey, 2013; Mercy & Steelman, 1982; P. Sammons et al., 2004). Second, literacy and numeracy abilities and deficits vary as a function of sex. In industrialised countries, there is a gender gap with girls outperforming boys in terms of reading, while girls often lag behind boys in mathematics (OECD, 2012). Indeed, male individuals are affected more often by specific reading difficulties (Lewis et al., 1994). However, while some authors demonstrated higher rates of girls with arithmetic impairments compared to boys (Moll, Kunze, et al., 2014), others suggested comparable prevalence rates for both sexes (Devine, Soltész, Nobes, Goswami, & Szűcs, 2013). Moreover, learning abilities and intellectual abilities are intrinsically linked. Per definition, specific literacy and numeracy impairments preclude a causal role of diminished intelligence for observed deficits (World Health Organization, 2018), and it has been suggested that genetic factors might have a larger impact in impaired individuals with higher IQ scores (Wadsworth, Olson, & DeFries, 2010).

Thus, when aiming to characterise specific contributions of neural systems to individual differences and deficits in either domain, a careful investigation and rigorous statistical control is necessary to identify effects unique to literacy or numeracy. This includes not only accounting for performance in the respective other domain, but equally important covariates such as measures of sociodemographic status or general intelligence. While evidence of comorbidity and confounds is plentiful, previous work frequently failed to include the large-scale psychometric and demographic testing needed to be able to comprehensively characterise their study sample. These vital oversights—for instance not investigating performance in mathematics when investigating literacy and vice versa – affect prominent neuroimaging studies of learning deficits (Ansari & Dhital, 2006; Clark et al., 2014; Hoeft et al., 2011; Hu et al., 2010; Kraft et al., 2016; Rotzer et al., 2009; B. A. Shaywitz et al., 2002; S. E. Shaywitz et al., 2003; Vandermosten et al., 2015) and typical development of both literacy (Ben-Shachar, Dougherty, Deutsch, & Wandell, 2011; Booth et al., 2004; Yeatman et al., 2012) and numeracy (Cho et al., 2011; Jolles, Supekar, et al., 2016; Rivera et al., 2005).

The empirical studies presented in this thesis (see Chapters 6 and 7) were designed to overcome the aforementioned shortcomings when investigating literacy deficits and numeracy development independently from each other. In both studies, neuroimaging measures were combined with comprehensive psychometric and demographic assessment, enabling a rigorous statistical control for prominent confounding factors such as general intelligence, sex, sociodemographic status as quantified by maternal education, in addition to early performance in reading, writing and mathematics.

CHAPTER 3

RESEARCH AIMS AND HYPOTHESES

The current research project was designed to analyse specific neural correlates of deficient literacy acquisition and individual differences in mathematical ability. As described in Chapter 2, previous literature associated regionally distinct brain development, both structurally as well as functionally, with differential literacy (Carreiras et al., 2009; Clark et al., 2014) and mathematical (Evans et al., 2015; Qin et al., 2014) ability. However, the comprehensive study of specific neural correlates of these higher cognitive skills faces several challenges that were only incompletely addressed by earlier research:

i. Longitudinal experimental designs are necessary to identify neurobiological profiles and developmental changes that are directly related to behavioural variation (see Section 2.1.2.2). Specifically, assessment of the respective biological underpinnings needs to start before formal instruction in either literacy or mathematics has begun. However, longitudinal neuroimaging work starting before school is sparse.

ii. Due to the considerable covariation between literacy or numeracy skills (see Section 2.3), both domains need to be considered when studying specific correlates of distinct abilities.

iii. Differential and atypical brain development on the microanatomical scale potentially induces variable structural and functional profiles. As will be described in detail in Chapter 4, early developmental processes include neuronal migration, maturation of synapses and glial cells like oligodendrocytes, as well as synaptic pruning. These have the potential to profoundly change the developing brain's appearance and functional networks. While previous work selectively focused on specfific measures, a more integrated approach combining various anatomical and functional dimensions (see Chapter 5) is needed to provide a comprehensive understanding of the emergence of complex cognitive abilities and their developmental trajectories.

The current research project was designed to overcome these prominent shortcomings of previous work. Specifically, I sought to comprehensively examine neural correlates of literacy and numeracy acquisition while addressing these challenges by relying on a longitudinal data set that combines structural T_1-weighted (T_1), diffusion-weighted (dMRI) and resting-state functional magnetic resonance imaging (rsfMRI) measurements with psychometric testing of the same children at kindergarten and school age. On this basis, we designed two studies to analyse specific neural correlates of deficient literacy acquisition and individual differences in mathematical ability.

3.1   EMPIRICAL STUDY I: UNRAVELING POTENTIAL CAUSES FROM CONSEQUENCES OF DEVELOPMENTAL DYSLEXIA

The aim of the first empirical study presented in this thesis was to identify neuronal correlates of developmental dyslexia (DD) and their development during the first two years of literacy acquisition. To this end, region of interest (ROI)-based comparisons of cortical grey matter anatomy, white matter structure and resting-state functional measures in dyslexic children and controls before and after literacy instruction were performed. Additionally, the predictive power of effects was assessed to test their ability for early prediction of DD.

As highlighted in Section 2.1.2.2, the gold-standard to disentangle potential causes from consequences of developmental disorders is to use longitudinal designs as presented in the current thesis. In particular, we investigated potential neural predispositions of DD by following children over several years from kindergarten to school, assessing their brain structure and resting-state functional development via magnetic resonance imaging (MRI). Concomitantly, participants' cognitive development was monitored via comprehensive psychometric testing. Critically, assessing individual's reading and writing skills at the end of second grade in school allowed us to compare cortical facets of children that have developed dyslexia later in life with typical controls prior to literacy acquisition, thereby removing the confound of impoverished literacy experience. Additionally, individual mathematical performance was included as a covariate in all statistical analyses, such that results can be ascribed specifically to literacy deficits independent of individual numeracy performance. Thus, we addressed the following main question:

- Which neural differences distinguish future dyslexic children from typically developing controls already prior to formal literacy instruction and after two years of schooling?

Hypothesis I.a   Following the literature currently available on preliterate children (Clark et al., 2014), we expected neural differences between dyslexic cases and controls to be confined to the phonological system. In particular, we anticipated replicating previous results indicating atypical functioning and structural organisation of left superior temporal regions, specifically the primary auditory cortex.

Hypothesis I.b   In line with post mortem work on adult dyslexic individuals reporting polymicrogyria within the left perisylvian cortex (Galaburda, LoTurco, Ramus, Fitch, & Rosen, 2006), we expected significantly increased gyrification of the left perisylvian cortex already in children as young as five years of age.

Hypothesis I.c   Beyond the sparse longitudinal work available pointing towards atypical structural organisation in confined regions associated with phonological processing, cross-sectional evidence and work on preliterate children as risk of literacy impairments suggest altered interregional connectivity in the dorsal reading network (see Section 2.1.1; Rimrodt, Peterson, Denckla, Kaufmann, & Cutting, 2010; Saygin et al., 2013; Skeide et al., 2015). In line with these reports, we hypothesised that atypical functional and structural connectivity of the dorsal reading network distinguish individuals with DD from controls both before and after literacy instruction. In particular, we assumed differences to appear in connections between superior temporal cortex areas such as the planum temporale and the primary auditory cortex and upstream prefrontal regions.

3.2 EMPIRICAL STUDY II: SURFACE PLASTICITY AND EARLY NUMERACY SKILLS

The aim of the second empirical study presented in this thesis was to characterise systematic relationships between developmental trajectories of brain structure and individual numeracy competence in typically developing children, independent of behavioural variability in literacy expertise. To this end, data from children who developed specific literacy impairments or who were at a familial risk for DD were not considered in this second study in order to exclude potential confounding effects. As pointed out in Section 2.2.1, previous research investigated the brain basis of magnitude processing in preschool children (Cantlon et al., 2006) and development of simple arithmetic skills in school-age participants (Qin et al., 2014; Rivera et al., 2005). However, little attention has been paid to neural correlates of emerging numeracy abilities during the first years of formal in-

struction when children move from approximate to exact calculation (Cho et al., 2011). Therefore, the current analysis focused
on exactly this age range, by quantifying cortical surface plasticity from kindergarten to second grade in school. Importantly,
I included measures beyond more traditional structural indices
like grey matter volume (GMV) or cortical thickness (CT) (Evans
et al., 2015; Rivera et al., 2005), also exploring gyrification, cortical folding complexity and sulcus depth. Thus, the following
main question was addressed:

- Which particular developmental trajectories of brain surface
  anatomy from kindergarten to primary school age are associated with individual numeracy attainment after two years
  of formal mathematical education?

Hypothesis II.a   We expected cortical plasticity to correlate
with individual differences in primary school numeracy ability
in regions associated with early magnitude and later arithmetic
processing, i. e. the intraparietal sulcus (IPS; Cantlon et al., 2006;
Jolles, Ashkenazi, et al., 2016) and the posterior parietal cortex
(PPC; Cantlon et al., 2006; Menon, 2010; Qin et al., 2014; Rivera
et al., 2005), and areas involved in arithmetic problem solving,
i. e. the prefrontal cortex (PFC; Cho et al., 2011; Evans et al.,
2015; Rivera et al., 2005) and medial temporal lobe (MTL; Cho
et al., 2011; Qin et al., 2014; Rivera et al., 2005; Supekar et al.,
2013).

Hypothesis II.b   For the parietal lobe specifically, we hypothesised a differential involvement of subregions for distinct

numeracy-related abilities, following the model of the PPC suggested by Dehaene et al. (2003). Specifically, we expected IPS
plasticity to be related to arithmetic processing and superior
parietal lobe (SPL) plasticity to be associated with visuospatial
magnitude processing.

CHAPTER 4

BRAIN STRUCTURAL AND FUNCTIONAL DEVELOPMENT

The human brain is a remarkably complex organ. Composed of approximately 85 billion neurons (Azevedo et al., 2009) with tens of thousands of synapses per cell (Cragg, 1975) and thus potentially over 100 trillion connections at the adult age, it is the origin of human thinking, action, memory, and consciousness. To fathom neural correlates of literacy and mathematical acquisition to be investigated in this thesis, one needs to understand the key principles governing brain development itself. This basic understanding is particularly important for identifying deviant brain maturation and its link to behavioural deficits and variation.

Thus, this chapter provides an overview of brain development in general and maturation of cortical structure in particular. After a brief introduction to the anatomy of the human cerebrum in Section 4.1, Section 4.2 describes general principles of cellular brain development in utero and across the lifespan. Section 4.3 highlights links between the micro- and the macroscopic scale, focusing on more global maturational changes in measures like cortical folding and thickness. Finally, Section 4.4 provides a brief overview of functional brain development.

4.1 GENERAL BRAIN STRUCTURE

The brain can be subdivided into several major structures. The largest of these is the cerebrum, which is composed of grey and white matter.

The outer mantle of the cerebrum, the cerebral cortex, is a highly folded, mutli-layered structure that consists of grey matter. Ranging between 2–5 mm in thickness, it houses different cellular structures, including the cell bodies of the brain's information processing cells, neurons (Stiles & Jernigan, 2010). From inside to outside, density and composition of cortical cell types vary, giving rise to a distinct laminar pattern. Across the cortex, individual layers show high structural variability, allowing for parcellations based on cytoarchitectonic composition (Brodmann, 1909; von Economo & Koskinas, 1925). Beyond these variations in structure, different cortical regions are selectively engaged in very specific cognitive functions such as processing linguistic syntax (Friederici, 2018), numerosity (Cantlon et al., 2006), or written words (Glezer et al., 2009).

Individual cortical areas are connected via neuronal projections that run beneath the grey matter mantle, forming the white matter. Its white appearance stems from myelin, a lipid-rich substance formed by a specific type of glial cell, so-called oligodendrocytes. Mature oligodendrocytes form few membranous outgrowths that spiral concentrically around nearby neuronal projections (Kandel, Barres, & Hudspeth, 2013). These tight sheaths provide the basis for saltatory conduction, thus greatly improving axonal conduction velocity (Fields et al., 2014). Importantly, functionally specific regions share variable afferent and efferent connectivity with other areas in the brain, giving rise to hierarchically organised networks (Park & Friston, 2013). In this way, the cerebral cortex ultimately supports complex higher cognitive abilities such as learning, memory, language, executive control and emotion (Kandel & Hudspeth, 2013).

4.2   MICROANATOMICAL BRAIN DEVELOPMENT

Development of the neural system begins with formation of the neural tube during the third week of gestation in utero (Stiles & Jernigan, 2010). Neural progenitors that can develop into all cell types of the future central nervous system line the inside of the neural tube (Jessell & Sanes, 2013). From there on, further development of the cortex can be divided into three crucial and partially overlapping processes: (a) neuronal division and migration, (b) development of neural connectivity, and (c) synaptogenesis and synaptic pruning (Budday, Steinmann, & Kuhl, 2015a).

Process (a), neuronal division and migration, starts after formation of the neural tube and is typically completed until the first half of gestation (Raybaud, Ahmad, Rastegar, Shroff, & Al Nassar, 2013). Neurons migrate from the neural plate in an 'inside-out' fashion. In effect, cells generated early during development form the innermost cortical layers, and later-formed neurons ultimately reside more adjacent to the pial surface (Stiles & Jernigan, 2010). The distinct 6-layered structure of neocortex becomes recognizable by gestational week 18 (Budday et al., 2015a).

Process (b) commences as soon as neurons reach their target position and begin to differentiate, sprouting dendrites and axons. Thus, the temporal trajectory of early brain connectivity parallels the 'inside-out' pattern of neuronal migration: deeper layers connect to subcortical targets before midgestation and superficial layers form intra-cortical, short association fibres and long-range cortico-cortical connections from gestational week 28 until after birth (Raybaud et al., 2013).

Process (c) is comprised of temporally overlapping stages of synapse formation and elimination. Widespread exuberant synaptogenesis (Innocenti & Price, 2005) occurs in concert with the growth of neuronal projections. This initial, large-scale formation of synapses starts before gestational week 27 (Huttenlocher & Dabholkar, 1997) and leads to a widespread surplus of transient synaptic connections (Innocenti & Price, 2005). It is characterised by highly heterogenous and heterochronous patterns throughout the cortex (Huttenlocher & Dabholkar, 1997), with prefrontal areas showing increases in synaptic density beyond four years of age (Liu et al., 2012). Concomitantly, elimination of synapses starts around the end of gestation and extends until mid-adolescence (Budday et al., 2015a; Huttenlocher & Dabholkar, 1997). During this period, exuberant projections and synapses generated early in cortical development are selectively eliminated, thereby refining the neural circuitry and establishing a more mature synaptic architecture (Neniskyte & Gross, 2017).

Despite the first appearance of sparse myelin in subcortical structures by gestational week 25 (Hasegawa et al., 1992), white matter development in utero is mainly characterised by pre-myelination processes. First oligodendrocyte progenitors form around gestational week 10 and need to undergo several stages before being transformed into myelin-forming cells (Barateiro & Fernandes, 2014). Unlike neural progenitor cells, immature oligodendrocytes travel considerable distances before arriving and proliferating at their target region within the white matter (Nave & Werner, 2014). After birth, the pace of myelination increases significantly and most rapidly during the first first year of life (Brody, Kinney, Kloman, & Gilles, 1987; Gao et al., 2009; Stiles & Jernigan, 2010). Akin to neuronal development, maturation of white matter is characterised by regional variations. Primary sensorimotor areas start getting myelinated after deep subcortical structures, followed by a systematic progression of white matter maturation in a posterior to anterior fashion (Brody et al., 1987; Hasegawa et al., 1992; Kinney, Brody, Kloman, & Gilles, 1988). After the first year of life, the rate of myelination decreases (Gao et al., 2009; Tau & Peterson, 2010) but generation and proliferation of oligodendrocytes, and thus myelination, persists throughout life (Stiles & Jernigan, 2010).

4.3 MACROANATOMICAL BRAIN DEVELOPMENT

The microanatomical development explained in the previous section is intrinsically linked to profound changes in the developing brain's macroanatomy that occur concomitantly.

Following a region-specific progression, development of cortical volume reflects the highly heterogenous and heterochronous pattern of cell maturation, proliferation, and pruning across the brain. Over development, there is a net decrease of total grey matter (Lebel & Beaulieu, 2011, see Figure 4.1). However, rigorous analysis of cortical volume maturation revealed a more complex developmental pattern. In a sample of 145 participants longitudinally assessed at approximately 2-year intervals, Lenroot and Giedd (2006) found that grey matter volume typically follows an inverted U shaped trajectory with region-specific peaks at different timepoints (see Figure 4.2).

A further crucial component of the cerebral surface anatomy is cortical thickness (CT), reflecting both dynamic developmental brain changes and neuroplasticity induced by experience. The pace of CT increase is most pronounced over the first year of life (Lyall et al., 2015). However, the exact developmental trajectory of cortical thickness maturation thereafter presents a matter of debate (Walhovd, Fjell, Giedd, Dale, & Brown, 2016).

Most early studies suggested a general developmental progression similar to the inverse U-shape observed for grey matter volume development. For instance, Shaw et al. (2008) reported a widespread pattern of initial CT increase across childhood, with

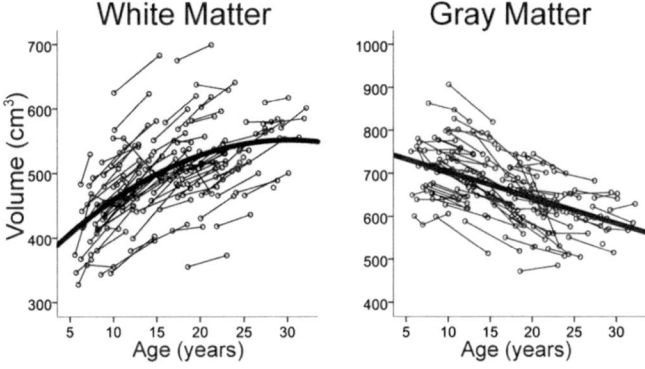

Figure 4.1: Developmental changes of white matter and grey matter volume from age 5-32 years, derived from 103 individuals. Reprinted from "Longitudinal Sevelopment of Human Brain Wiring Continues from Childhood into Adulthood" by C. Lebel and C. Beaulieu, 2011, *Journal of Neuroscience, 31(30)*, p. 10939. Copyright 2011 by the authors. Reproduced with permission of SOCIETY FOR NEUROSCIENCE in the format Republish in a thesis/dissertation via Copyright Clearance Center.

regionally specific peaks reached at different time points, followed by subsequent decline throughout adolescence and adulthood, in occipital, parietal, lateral frontal, lateral temporal, anterior cingulate and insular cortex (see Figure 4.3). A linear progression of consistent cortical thinning was only observed in restricted, mostly medially located regions. These results support previous literature describing such a pattern of age-dependent growth and decrease of CT (Shaw et al., 2007; Shaw et al., 2006; Sowell et al., 2004).

In contrast, a series of more recent studies has indicated a continuous global reduction in grey matter thickness across childhood (Kharitonova, Martin, Gabrieli, & Sheridan, 2013), extending into adolescence and adulthood (Amlien et al., 2016; T. T. Brown & Jernigan, 2012; T. T. Brown et al., 2012; Ducharme et

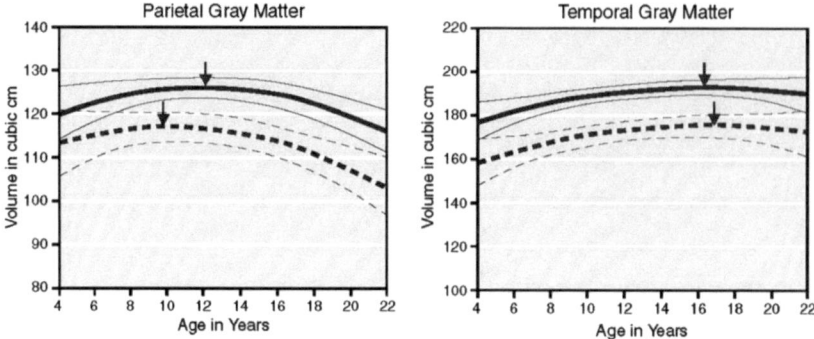

Figure 4.2: Age-dependent inverse U-shaped trajectories of grey matter volume in parietal and temporal cortex, derived from 145 individuals. The bold solid line indicates the progression of grey matter volume in male and bold dotted lines the trajectory in female individuals. Light solid and dotted lines denote the respective 95% confidence intervals. Arrows indicate age of peak volume. Adapted from "Brain Development in Children and Adolescents: Insights from Anatomical Magnetic Resonance Imaging" by R. K. Lenroot and J. N. Giedd, 2006, *Neuroscience & Biobehavioral Reviews, 30*, p. 724. Copyright 2006 by Elsevier Ltd. Adapted with permission.

al., 2016; O'Donnell, Noseworthy, Levine, & Dennis, 2005, c.f. Figure 4.4). For example, Ducharme et al. (2016) examined the developmental tracjectory of CT between the ages of 4.9 and 22 years and identified widespread patterns of linear thinning throughout the cortex. Crucially, when their analysis was more stringently controlled for data quality, almost all areas in the brain exhibited clear linear patterns of cortical thinning across age.

Such critical inconsistencies regarding CT trajectories reported in structural neuroimaging studies are difficult to reconcile. As pointed out by Walhovd et al. (2016), it is important to note that not just demographic factors of the target population

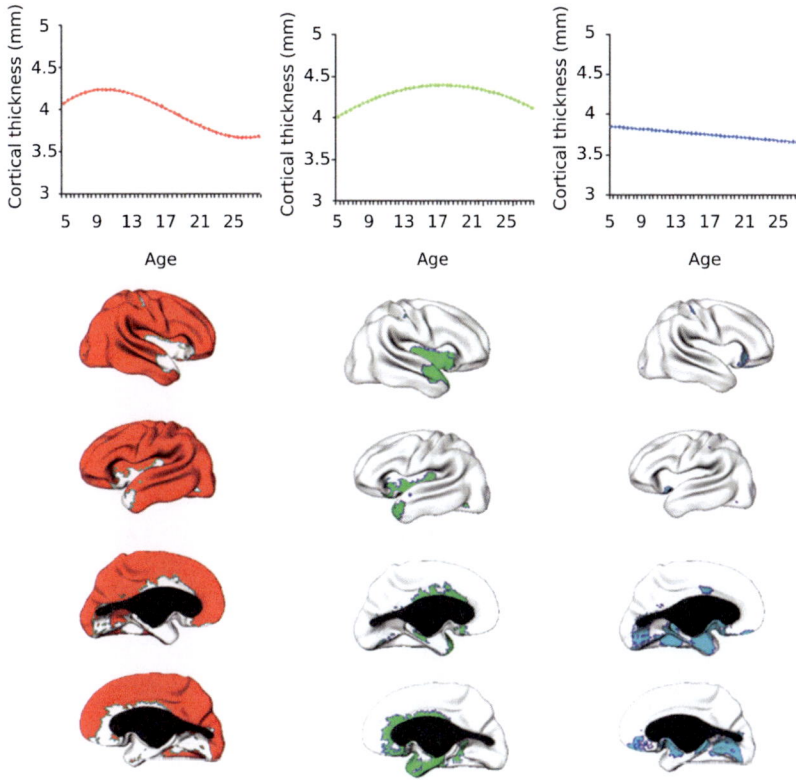

Figure 4.3: Regions characterised by variable developmental trajectories of cortical thickness development, based on MRI data from 375 individuals. Red and green regions are marked by a pattern of initial thickness increase and subsequent decline, while regions in blue show a linear rate of thinning. Adapted from "Neurodevelopmental Trajectories of the Human Cerebral Cortex" by P. Shaw et al., 2008, *Journal of Neuroscience, 28(14)*, p. 3588. Copyright 2008 by Society for Neuroscience. Reproduced with permission of SOCIETY FOR NEUROSCIENCE in the format Republish in a thesis/dissertation via Copyright Clearance Center.

but also methodological choices may have a crucial impact on assessment of CT development.

Cortical thickness systematically covaries with the laminar structure of the cortex (von Economo & Koskinas, 1925; Wagstyl, Ronan, Goodyer, & Fletcher, 2015). However, it is important to

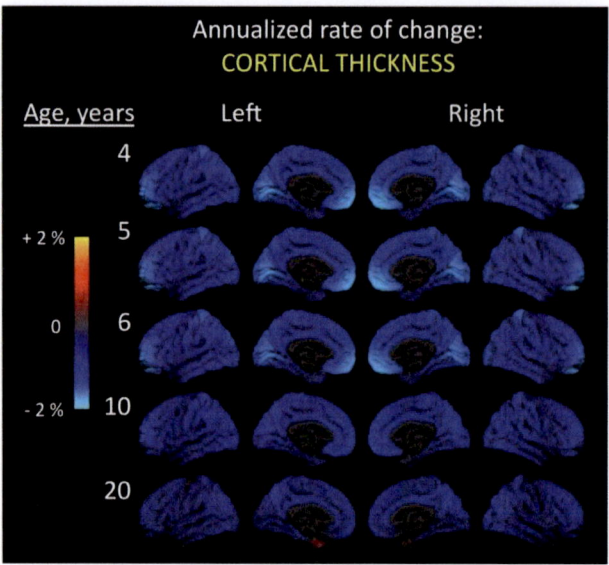

Figure 4.4: Rate of change of cortical thickness across the brain for different age groups, derived from 202 individuals aged 4-20 years. Reprinted from "Brain Development During the Preschool Years" by T. T. Brown and T. L. Jernigan, 2012, *Neuropsychology Review, 22(4),* p. 318. Copyright 2012 by Springer Nature. Reprinted with permission.

note that cortical thickness is not a biomarker of neuronal density per se (Skoglund, Pascher, & Berthold, 1996). La Fougère et al. (2011) described an inconsistent relationship between neuron count and cortical thickness in a combined PET-MRI study: thickness was independent of cell number in prefrontal and inferior parietal areas, and even inversely related to neuronal density in temporal, occipital, primary sensory, and motor cortices. Therefore, CT has to be interpreted with care and may instead be related to more general elements of cytoarchitecture, specifically axons, dendrites and synapses (Wagstyl & Lerch, 2018). A further methodological issue concerns the possible interaction of grey matter and white matter in MRI. Increased intracortical myelin content enhances the white matter signal and potentially compromises the grey matter signal. Thus, results of cortical thinning might in fact be a marker of progressive myelination of deep cortical white matter rather than changes in the thickness of the cortical sheath itself (Natu et al., 2018; Stiles & Jernigan, 2010).

While the trajectory of CT is still debated, the development of cortical gyrification pattens is less controversial. In concert with developing connectivity, the cortex begins to fold (Raybaud et al., 2013). Primary sulci like the sylvian, central and inferior frontal fissures form until gestational week 26, followed by development of secondary sulci starting throughout prenatal week 30 and tertiary sulci starting during gestational week 36 (Stiles & Jernigan, 2010). While the location of primary sulci is remarkably consistent across individuals (Lohmann, von Cramon, & Colchester, 2008), secondary and tertiary foldings show more variability (Bartley, Jones, & Weinberger, 1997). Importantly, to date, debate continues about the underlying key mechanisms driving cortical folding (Bayly, Taber, & Kroenke, 2014).

For instance, the axonal tension hypothesis posits that folding is induced through physical strain along axons connecting cortical regions, thereby drawing them together such that the cortex bulges outward (Van Essen, 1997). This view is consistent with principles of efficient wiring, since reducing the projection length also minimises the conduction time. However, G. Xu et al. (2010) failed to show significant axonal tension in the centre of developing gyri, challenging this account.

Others associated the onset of cortical folding with the complex interplay of radial and tangential cortical proliferation (Bayly, Okamoto, Xu, Shi, & Taber, 2013; Bayly et al., 2014; Tallinen et al., 2016), spatially and temporally heterogenous growth patterns (Bayly et al., 2014; Budday & Steinmann, 2018; Ronan et al., 2014; G. Xu et al., 2010; T. Zhang et al., 2016), developmental trajectories of cortical thickness (Budday, Raybaud, & Kuhl, 2014; Tallinen et al., 2016), as well as variable properties concerning elasticity and stiffness of grey and white matter (Budday & Steinmann, 2018; Tallinen et al., 2016; T. Zhang et al., 2016).

In stark contrast to the remarkable variability of grey matter thickness and volume across the life-span, cortical folding is much more stable (Armstrong, Schleicher, Omran, Curtis, & Zilles, 1995). Li et al. (2014) demonstrated the most rapid postnatal changes in cortical folding during the first year of life, followed by a decreasing rate of change (see Figure 4.5). Thus, not just the pattern of primary, but also that of secondary and tertiary gyrification seems to be determined within the very first years of life. Consequently, while differences in folding patterns have also been linked to ongoing myelination and synaptic remodeling (Blanton et al., 2001), they are often taken as a sensitive marker for deviant pre- and early postnatal neural development (Bayly et al., 2014; Mutlu et al., 2013). For instance, Schaer et al. (2009) identified deviant gyrification in patients with a neurogenetic disorder that is frequently associated with abberant neuronal migration and proliferation.

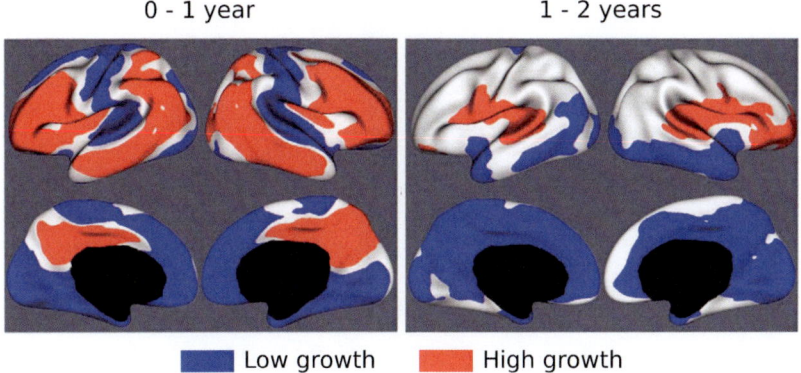

Figure 4.5: Significant clusters of change in cortical gyrification within the first (left) and second (right) year of life, derived from 73 longitudinally assessed infants. Clusters are divided into regions with high growth rates (red) and regions with significant, yet low growth rates. Adapted from "Mapping Longitudinal Development of Local Cortical Gyrification in Infants from Birth to 2 Years of Age" by G. Li et al., 2014, *Journal of Neuroscience, 34(12)*, p. 4234. Copyright 2014 by the authors. Reproduced with permission of SOCIETY FOR NEUROSCIENCE in the format Republish in a thesis/dissertation via Copyright Clearance Center.

In line with molecular observations of continuous oligodendrocyte generation and proliferation throughout life, Lebel and Beaulieu (2011) report a steady longitudinal increase in whole brain white matter volume from five years until 32 years of age (see Figure 4.1). A similar trajectory of white matter maturation has been described by Barnea-Goraly et al. (2005), who not only found sustained changes in white matter density with age, but also specific age-related increases in white matter anisotropy in individuals aged six to 20 years. Hence, over development from childhood until adulthood, myelin progressively accumulates in a highly organised, coherent fashion along axons and fibre tracts.

4.4   FUNCTIONAL BRAIN DEVELOPMENT

Much like the anatomical changes described in Sections 4.2 and 4.3, functional brain development is a highly dynamic process. As neurons mature and form new connections, they also start transmitting signals from one cell to another. These processes give rise to first functional networks that can already be identified in utero (Schöpf, Kasprian, Brugger, & Prayer, 2012; Thomason et al., 2013). Remarkably, a range of functional circuits is already in place by term (Doria et al., 2010), most prominently encompassing primary sensory and motor regions (Fransson et al., 2007; Lin et al., 2008). Further during subsequent development, the proportion of brain volume that is part of these networks increases over the first few years of life, following regionally specific trajectories (Lin et al., 2008). During childhood, functional interactions between regions exhibit more and more adult-like patterns. In children six to seven years of age, primary visual, auditory, somatosensory and frontoparietal networks spatially resemble adult cortical networks, while others associated with executive control and attention show less mature profiles (Thornburgh et al., 2017). Further throughout adolescence until adulthood, individual networks mature, becoming increasingly independent from each other and, thereby, functionally specific (Stevens, Pearlson, & Calhoun, 2009).

Considering stimulus- or task-related processing, a similar shift from diffuse to functionally specific activity can be observed. For instance, infants show a considerably broader tuning of electrophysiological responses in word learning (Neville, Mills, & Lawson, 1992) or face recognition (de Haan, Pascalis, & Johnson, 2002) than exhibited by adults. With age or stimulus experience, more specialised functioning emerges (Johnson, 2001). For instance, functional activation during a cognitive control task is still widespread in nine-year-old children, and becomes more focal in task-relevant regions throughout the next three years of life (Durston et al., 2006). Importantly, these functional responses as well as the functional networks described above are highly plastic and may be shaped by individual experiences and skill acquisition. For instance, already brief phoneme-grapheme training enhances the activity within the fusiform gyrus in six-year-old, pre-reading children, reflecting how this specific brain region tunes to print (Brem et al., 2010). Not just during development, but also throughout later life, the brain remains plastic, as demonstrated e. g. by functional reorganisation following motor skill learning in adults (Karni et al., 1998).

CHAPTER 5

EXAMINING BRAIN STRUCTURE AND FUNCTION
VIA MAGNETIC RESONANCE IMAGING

As outlined in Chapter 3, the current thesis aims to provide a comprehensive analysis of potential neural correlates of literacy impairment and numeracy development. To this end, the analyses presented here combine measures of literacy and mathematical ability with various estimates of structural and functional brain development assessed via magnetic resonance imaging (MRI). Importantly, a fundamental understanding of the basic principles underlying this neuroimaging approach is key to interpret MRI data. Therefore, this chapter initially provides information about the foundations of MRI measurements (Sections 5.1 and 5.2).

Furthermore, sophisticated imaging processing techniques are necessary to derive specific information of neuroanatomical and neurofunctional measures from the basic output of an MRI machine. Based on these techniques, it is possible to draw conclusions about grey matter (GM) volume and thickness, cortical surface geometry such as gyrification, sulcus depth and cortical folding complexity, white matter (WM) structure, functional connectivity between regions, regional functional homogeneity and fractional amplitude of low frequency fluctuations of the resting brain. As described in Chapter 4, these aspects show characteristic changes during development, relate to cognitive processing and may be reflective more fundamental maturational processes shaping the brain. To create a fundamental understanding of these MRI-derived measures, the remainder of this chapter gives detailed accounts describing how GM (Section 5.3), WM (Section 5.4) and resting-state functional properties (Section 5.5) can be obtained from imaging data.

5.1 MAGNETIC RESONANCE IMAGING

MRI proved a valuable tool for analysing the composition and structure as well as functional properties of the brain. Prior to the advent of MRI, estimation of neuroanatomy relied on effortful histology work on post-mortem samples. Investigation of functional properties was restricted to animal and lesion models. With respect to developmental research specifically, MRI data provides the basis for determining rate and change of differential regional brain maturation between individuals and groups. Thus, this non-invasive, full-brain imaging approach offers insights into the relation between the maturation of both the brain's functional and structural organisation and cognitive development (Casey, Tottenham, Liston, & Durston, 2005; Gilmore, Knickmeyer, & Gao, 2018; Kanai & Rees, 2011; Lebel & Deoni, 2018). For instance, MRI techniques allowed to shed light onto associations of GM growth and higher-order cognitive functioning (Breukelaar et al., 2017). Furthermore, the importance of white matter development of tracts connecting temporoparietal and inferior frontal regions for the emergence of theory of mind (Grosse Wiesmann, Schreiber, Singer, Steinbeis, & Friederici, 2017) and complex language abilities (Skeide, Brauer, & Friederici, 2016) was revealed by diffusion–weighted magnetic resonance imaging (dMRI).

5.1.1 *Basic principles of magnetic resonance imaging measurements*

As a component of water molecules, hydrogen is one of the most abundant atoms in the human body. The nucleus of each hydrogen atom contains a single proton that spins around its axis, producing a small magnetic field. MRI exploits this inherent magnetic property of protons. During an MRI measurement, the scanner exerts a strong, static external magnetic field B_0 on the body. As a result, the hydrogen atoms align to this field, such that the contained protons spin – or precess – around their axis, creating longitudinal magnetisation (i. e.net magnetisation along the direction of B_0; Westbrook & Talbot, 2019). The angular frequency of this precession movement is known as the Larmor frequency ω_0. It grows in direct proportion to (a) the strength of the B_0 field and (b) the gyromagnetic ratio γ, a constant specific to a particular nucleus, relating its magnetic momentum to its angular momentum (B. M. Dale, Brown, & Semelka, 2015):

$$\omega_0 = \gamma B_0. \tag{5.1}$$

In MRI, the proton frequency distribution is additionally influenced by secondary magnetic fields generated by gradient coils that focally distort the primary B_0. These coils are commonly arranged perpendicular to each other in three directions (i. e.x, y, and z). Induced frequency changes vary depending of the position of a nucleus along the gradient directions, thus allowing for spatial encoding of magnetic resonance recordings to produce sagittal, coronal and axial images, respectively (Lauterbur, 1973).

Radiofrequency (RF) coils in an MRI scanner transmit pulses and receive signals during a measurement. Specifically, an induced RF pulse generates a second magnetic field B_1 perpendicular to the stationary B_0, oscillating at the specific ω_0 of the current system. Consequently, the proton alignment is disturbed in two ways: (a) a proportion of protons flip to a high-energy state, thereby decreasing longitudinal magnetisation and (b) protons become synchronised, precessing in phase. As a result, the net magnetisation of the whole system is shifted perpendicularly to the B_0 field, generating so-called transverse magnetisation. After the RF pulse is switched off, the protons gradually resume their original, de-phased state along the B_0 field (Westbrook & Talbot, 2019).

During this period, the net magnetisation in direction of B_0 increases over time, resulting in so-called T_1-relaxation (red curve in Figure 5.1). Conversely, as the protons return to a more desynchronised state, magnetisation into the transverse direction decreases, known as transverse or T_2-relaxation (light blue curve in

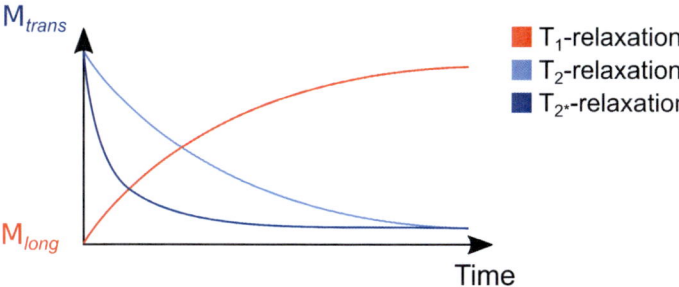

Figure 5.1: Schematic illustration of T_1-, T_2- and T_{2^*}-relaxation over time. M_{long} = longitudinal magnetisation (in the direction of the B_0 field); M_{trans} = transversal magnetisation (perpendicular to the B_0 field).

Figure 5.1). This dephasing of spins is additionally accelerated by inhomogeneities of the primary magnetic field. Therefore, the observed transverse relaxation essentially consists of a combination of T_2-relaxation and said inhomogeneities, termed T_{2^*} (dark blue curve in Figure 5.1; B. M. Dale et al., 2015).

Importantly, protons emit the energy absorbed from the RF pulse during relaxation, creating a transient Nuclear Magnetic Resonance (NMR) signal (Bloch, Hansen, & Packard, 1946; Purcell, Torrey, & Pound, 1946) detectable as induced currents in the RF coils of the MRI set up. Importantly, organic tissue such as the brain is characterised by heterogeneous proton density distributions due to the different composition of cells and variable proportions of hydrogen atoms. These characteristic differences cause distinct relaxation rates for different tissue types. If movement of water molecules is less restricted as e. g.in the cerebrospinal fluid (CSF), their protons require more time to leave the high-energy state, thus T_1-relaxation proceeds at a slower rate. Reversely, in regions with more restricted water movement, for instance due to the high-lipid protein myelin in white matter, T_1-relaxation is quicker. For T_{2^*} imaging, the reverse pattern holds at a much quicker rate (Westbrook & Talbot, 2019).

Different MRI sequences capture these distinct relaxation rates—and thus the contrast between different tissue structures (see Figure 5.3)—by choice of appropriate imaging parameters. Specifically, T_1 and T_{2^*} imaging capture the longitudinal relaxation and transversal relaxation rates, respectively. These signal values are converted into a temporary image space, so-called k-space, storing a digitised version during data acquisition. After applying a Fourier transform, the final MRI image in 3D dimensional space is obtained with information of relaxation rate at a specific x-, y- and z-position stored in a volumetric pixel, a voxel (McRobbie, Moore, Graves, & Prince, 2017).

5.1.2   *Parameters determining image contrast*

The exact whole-brain MRI scanning routine depends on the specific sequence applied. Due to their specificity, each technique employs different values for measurement parameters. For the sake of this thesis, the effects of choosing different measurement parameters are highlighted based on the example of a typical gradient echo imaging sequence (Elster, 1993), as the basis of the magnetisation-prepared 2 rapid acquisition gradient echo sequence (MP2RAGE; Marques et al., 2010) used to acquire the structural images for the studies presented in Chapters 6 and 7.

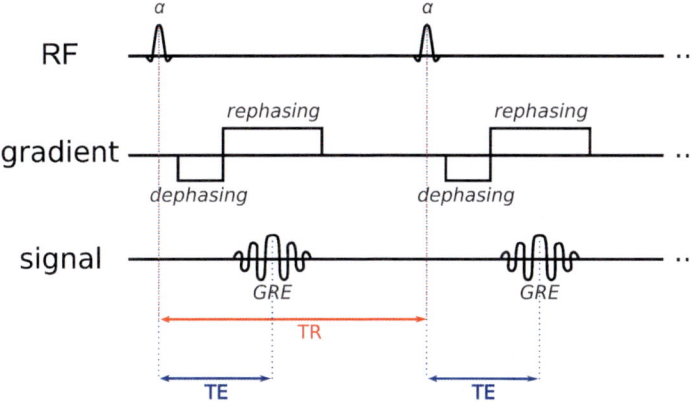

Figure 5.2: The basic gradient echo imaging sequence. RF = radiofrequency pulse; α = flip angle; GRE = gradient echo; TR =
repetition time; TE = echo time.

During gradient echo imaging, a series of RF pulses is applied at a certain flip angle α at equidistant time intervals. These
pulses excite a single slice of brain tissue (see Figure 5.2). The
time intervals between them are referred to as repetition time
(TR). The more time elapses between two pulses, the more protons within different types of tissue—even the more slowly relax-
ating CSF—fully regain longitudinal relaxation before the next
pulse. If all tissues are fully relaxated, they will emmit comparable signals, and image contrast driven by longitudinal relaxation will be low. If, however, the TR is short, tissue that is more
strongly longitudinally relaxated releases stronger signals, while
tissue with lower levels of magnetisation into the direction of the
B_0 field emits weaker signals. Hence, this procedure makes the
characteristic longitudinal relaxation time differences between
tissues detectable (Westbrook & Talbot, 2019). In this way, the
T1-contrast of the image is modulated (see bottom left in Figure 5.3).

Subsequent to each RF pulse, a pair of dephasing and rephasing gradients is applied, producing the gradient echo signal that is ultimately sampled during the scan. The time between the centre of the RF pulse and the readout of said signal is the echo time (TE; McRobbie et al., 2017). By choosing an appropriate TE, the T_2^*-contrast of the final image is modulated. If TE is low, spins—independent of the type of tissue they reside in—are given little time to go out of phase. Consequently, the emitted signal will not be influenced by the specific differences in T_2^*-relaxation times, thereby having little T_2^*-weighting. Only if a longer TE is chosen, the distinct differences in transversal magnetisation decay will have an effect on the final signal, obtaining a T_2^*-weighted contrast (Westbrook & Talbot, 2019).

In summary, T_1 images are typically acquired with short TR and TE, while long values for TR and TE are chosen for T_2^* imaging (see Figure 5.3). Consequently, the choice of these parameters critically determines the contrast of the resulting images, i. e. the difference in terms of signal strength obtained from different tissue types. Thus, depending on the image weighting, conclusions about in vivo tissue characteristics can be drawn.

5.2   FUNCTIONAL MAGNETIC RESONANCE IMAGING

Beyond studying anatomy, MRI is able to capture functional properties of the brain. A functional scan relies on the fact that the magnetic properties of haemoglobin—the respiratory protein of red blood cells—vary dependent on its state of oxy-

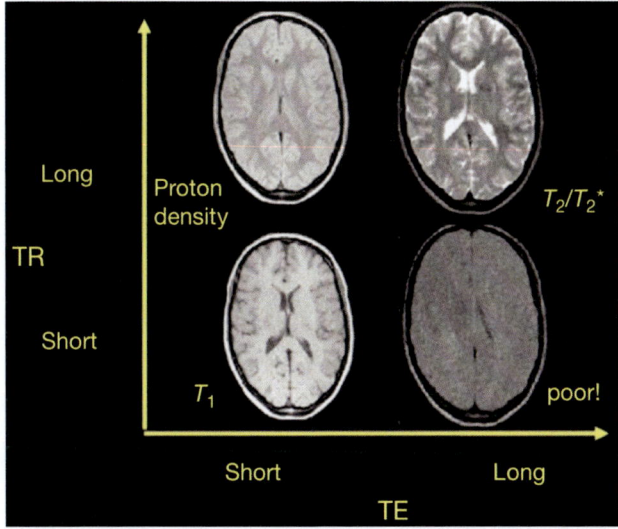

Figure 5.3: Examples of MRI contrast weightings in relation to the choice of repetition time (TR) and echo time (TE). Bottom left: A T1-weighted image is obtained by choosing short values for both TR and TE. Consequently, CSF appears dark and WM appears light. Top right: To create T2- or T2*-weighted images, long TR and TE values are necessary. The CSF appears dark and WM appears light. Reprinted from "Anatomical MRI for human brain morphometry" (p.14), by A. van der Kouwe, B. Fischl, 2015. In A. W. Toga (Ed.), *Brain mapping: An encyclopedic reference*, 2015, San Diego, CA, USA: Academic Press: Elsevier. Copyright 2015 by Elsevier Inc. Reprinted with permission.

genation (Pauling & Coryell, 1936). When neurons become active, their oxygen consumption increases together the volume of deoxygenated blood. Due to its paramagnetic nature, deoxygenated haemoglobin induces inhomogeneities in the local magnetic field, enhancing the dephasing of proton spins and thereby leading to more rapid T_{2^*}-relaxation. Subsequently, the blood flow in the brain's microvasculature increases to supply active cells with new oxygen, diluting the concentration of deoxyhaemoglobin. Thus, the abundance of diamagnetic, oxygenated blood restores the homogeneity of the magnetic field again, consequently inducing an enhanced T_{2^*} signal (Deichmann, 2016). The characteristic trajectory of the initial small decrease and subsequent increase in T_{2^*} signal is captured using the so-called blood oxygenation level dependent (BOLD) contrast.

The relationship between the BOLD responses and neural activity have been investigated in animals and humans (Logothetis, Pauls, Augath, Trinath, & Oeltermann, 2001; Mukamel, 2005). For instance, in a seminal study, Logothetis et al. (2001) simultaneously performed fMRI while recording from electrodes in the visual cortex of monkeys, demonstrating the correspondence between the BOLD response and the pooled local field activity.

During fMRI measurements, a sequence of images that quantify the oxygenation patterns across time is obtained, reflecting changes in neural activity within a given voxel. In task-related fMRI, these signal changes are related to experimental manipulations. The functional focus of this thesis, however, lies in resting-state fMRI (rsfMRI), i. e.examining the brain's functional responses during rest. By relating spontaneous fluctuations of fMRI time series of regions, measures of functional coherence can be obtained. Consequently, this procedure allows for conclusions about brain networks even in the absence of a task (see Section 5.5).

5.3   EXAMINING GREY MATTER STRUCTURE

As discussed in Section 4.3, the cortical ribbon undergoes profound macroanatomical changes during development. Early in-

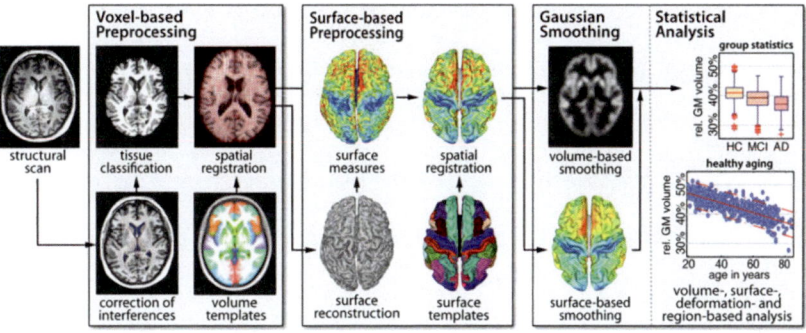

Figure 5.4: Preprocessing of structural MRI data for voxel- and surface-based morphometry. Images preprocessed within the voxel-based pipeline serve as basis for the surface-based reconstructions. Both voxel- and surface-based analyses require alignment to a template image or mesh, respectively. Final smoothing enhanced statistical sensitivity and renders data are more normally distributed. Adapted from "Surface and shape analysis" by R. Dahnke and C. Gaser, in G. Spalletta, F. Piras and T. Gili (Eds.), *Brain morphometry* (p. 58), 2018, New York, U.S.A.: Humana Press. Copyright 2018 by Springer Nature. Adapted with permission.

vestigations were restricted to laboursome post-mortem manual measures to gain insights about dynamic cortical maturation (Huttenlocher & Dabholkar, 1997). MRI extends the possibilities with non-invasive, in vivo approaches such as voxel-based (Ashburner & Friston, 2000) and surface-based morphometry (Dahnke, Yotter, & Gaser, 2013; A. M. Dale, Fischl, & Sereno, 1999; Fischl, Sereno, & Dale, 1999), highlighted in the following sections.

5.3.1 *Voxel-based morphometry*

Voxel–based morphometry (VBM; Ashburner & Friston, 2000; Mechelli, Price, Friston, & Ashburner, 2005) is an approach to quantify focal differences in GM structure from T_1-weighted

MRI data. Initial VBM preprocessing (see left side of Figure 5.4) involves alignment of the anatomical data with a standard brain template. In this way, macroscopic differences in size and structure of individual brains are compensated for. Consequently, only local variances in GM will be identified by the ensuing statistical analysis.

Registration to standard adult templates yields admissible results for data drawn from adult populations. However, such an alignment might introduce distortions in data derived from samples with more variable structural characteristics like children or patients (Yoon, Fonov, Perusse, Evans, & Brain Development Cooperative Group, 2009). Paediatric templates derived from equivalent age groups (Fonov, Evans, McKinstry, Almli, & Collins, 2009) or from the sample under investigation (Reuter, Schmansky, Rosas, & Fischl, 2012) circumvent this issue, as they reflect the region- and age-specific variations of the respective study group (see Chapter 4).

Next, images are segmented into different tissue classes (Ashburner & Friston, 2005). The segmentation algorithm applied in the empirical studies presented in Chapters 6 and 7 of this thesis relies on prior information provided as tissue probability maps (Ashburner & Friston, 1997). As with the initial image registration step, the use of age-appropriate priors is vital to ensure proper brain extraction.

In the final preprocessing step, spatially normalised and segmented GM images are smoothed using a volume-based kernel. As a result, the impact of local registration errors is attenuated and statistical sensitivity is enhanced. Furthermore, smoothed data are more normally distributed which is an essential prerequisite for statistical analysis (Lerch & Evans, 2005; Mechelli et al., 2005; S. M. Smith et al., 2006).

The VBM procedure as explained above generates maps of GM volume. It has been prominantly used to investigate GM structure in the context of developmental learning disorders such as DD (Richlan et al., 2013; Silani et al., 2005) and developmental dyscalculia (Rotzer et al., 2008), learning induced plasticity (Draganski et al., 2004; Draganski et al., 2006), and ageing (Hoffstaedter et al., 2015; Tisserand et al., 2004). However, disentangling the biological underpinnings driving changes in the measure of cortical volume is not trivial. For instance, GM volume quantified by VBM might not detect subtle changes differentially driven by CT and folding (Mechelli et al., 2005).

5.3.2 *Surface-based morphometry*

Surface-based techniques extend the possibilities of image analysis provided by VBM, enabling a detailed study of macroanatomical morphometric measures. For instance, surface–based morphometry (SBM) allows to examine CT and folding. Prominent software tools performing automatic surface reconstruction are the FreeSurfer image analysis suite (Fischl, 2012; FreeSurfer, 2014) and the Computational Anatomy Toolbox (CAT12; Gaser & Dahnke, 2017) for SPM12 (Friston, Ashburner, Kiebel, Nichols, & Penny, 2007).

Surface-based processing relies on initial, voxel-based preprocessing steps including segmentation and registration to a template (Dahnke & Gaser, 2018, see Section 5.3.1 and middle portion of Figure 5.4). Subsequently, surface reconstructions are generated from the volumetric MRI data as surface meshes, tessellated into triangular faces that connect individual cortical points designated by vertices (see Figure 5.4; Dahnke & Gaser, 2018; Fischl, 2012). Since the interface between GM and WM is often sharper than the borderline between GM and CSF, most approaches initially reconstruct the surface of the WM. This initial estimation is subsequently grown out in a bottom-up fashion, optimised and deformed to reconstruct the outer, pial surface of the brain (A. M. Dale et al., 1999; Kim et al., 2005; Tosun et al., 2004). To ensure comparability, individual surface meshes are spatially registered to a template mesh, commonly a sphere. Thus, when aligned, the individual data match in a vertex-by-vertex fashion.

Lastly, surface-based smoothing yields advantages comparable to those of the volume-based smoothing during VBM, such as enhancing statistical sensitivity and rendering data are more normally distributed (Lerch & Evans, 2005).

5.3.2.1 *Cortical thickness*

The thickness of the cortical ribbon is estimated as the distance between the segmented white matter and the pial surface. The method employed in the current thesis uses an automated procedure that combines surface and thickness estimation in one step (Dahnke et al., 2013), concomitantly diminishing area distortion and topological defects (Yotter, Dahnke, Thompson, & Gaser, 2011; Yotter, Thompson, & Gaser, 2011).

As described in Chapter 4.3, there is a systematic change of CT in different areas during development (Ducharme et al., 2016; Lyall et al., 2015; Shaw et al., 2008). Due to the inconsistent relationship between neuron count and CT (la Fougère et al., 2011; Skoglund et al., 1996) thickness variations assessed via MRI has been related to microanatomical processes like neuro-, glio- and synaptogenesis as well as synaptic pruning (Zatorre, Fields, & Johansen-Berg, 2012). Furthermore, decreases of CT during development may be a marker of progressive myelination of deep cortical layers (Natu et al., 2018).

5.3.2.2 *Gyrification index and cortical folding complexity*

Cortical gyrification is one of the most distinctive macroanatomical features of the brain. In the current thesis, its degree and developmental change were assessed using two separate measures, i. e. the gyrification index (GI) assessing local and cortical folding complexity (CF) assessing global gyrification, respectively.

The GI is defined as the absolute mean curvature along the highly convolved brain surface (Lüders et al., 2006). For this, a vector pointing outwards perpendicularly to the surface is defined for each vertex along the mesh. Subsequently, the absolute mean change of these vectors within the neighbourhood of a specified vertex is computed. Thus, the GI increases with increasing magnitude and frequency of folding, quantifying local gyrification.

CF is defined as the so-called fractal dimension of the individual points along the surface mesh. Theoretically, perfect fractal structures consist of an infinite number of self-similar shapes at different scales. Analysis of the fractal dimension in neuroimaging exploits the fact that the brain's surface structure exhibits some self-similarity, e. g. in terms of gyral profiles (Hofman, 2012). The method employed in this thesis to estimate the fractal dimension—and thus, the cortical folding complexity— uses a set of spherical harmonics basis functions to reconstruct the surface mesh representing cortex (Yotter, Nenadic, Ziegler, Thompson, & Gaser, 2011). From these functions, the number of self-similar shapes $N(l)$ can be derived and subsequently related to their smallest width l, yielding:

$$CF = \frac{log(N(l))}{log(1/l)}. \tag{5.2}$$

From this definition it follows that CF decreases with the number of self-similar shapes of decreasingly narrow widths. In this way, small CF values indicate more regular structural patterns. Thus, in terms of gyrification, CF quantifies how regular cortex is folded, providing insights into the more global cortical geometry.

As highlighted in Section 4.3, cortical gyrification is characterised by dynamic changes especially during early brain development. An increasing degree of cortical folding implies an increased surface area and thus increased GM volume, even if the level of CT remains constant morphological variations might be caused by diverging trajectories of neuronal growth or CT (Budday et al., 2014). In a longitudinal study tracing age-specific changes throughout childhood from six to 16 years, Blanton et al. (2001) linked the observed developmental trajectories to processes like ongoing myelination and synaptic remodeling. Importantly, systematic variations in the degree of cortical folding have been associated with cognitive functioning (Im, Raschle, Smith, Ellen Grant, & Gaab, 2016; Lüders et al., 2008).

5.3.2.3   *Sulcus depth*

Beyond frequency and regularity of foldings, another cortical surface feature is the sulcus depth (SD). This measure quantifies the inward Euclidean distance between the external brain surface and the banks of the sulcal grooves (Jones, Buchbinder, & Aharon, 2000).

Due to the highly convolved structure of the cortex, a certain proportion of the brain's surface is buried within the sulci (Armstrong et al., 1995). Importantly, regions with deeper sulci have a larger cortical surface area and thus increased GM volume independent of CT.

5.4   EXAMINING WHITE MATTER STRUCTURE

Next to the analysis of GM properties, MRI provides functionality to examine maturation and structure of the brain's WM. Specific MRI sequences allow for the generation of so-called dMRI.

5.4.1   *Diffusion–weighted magnetic resonance imaging*

The physical basis of diffusion–weighted magnetic resonance
imaging rests upon the idea of deriving WM information from
the proportion and directionality of water diffusion occurring
within. If located in an unrestricted liquid medium, water
molecules move freely and randomly, termed Brownian motion. In biological tissue, however, the surrounding cell structures interfere with this random motion (Le Bihan et al., 2001).
Specifically, certain tissue components like the neuronal cy-
toskeleton restrict diffusion into a specific direction. Thus, undi-
rected isotropic molecular movement is disturbed and becomes
anisotropic. In the brain, for instance, diffusion is more likely to
occur along white matter tracts than perpendicular to them. The
strength and directionality of this resulting anisotropy allows for
conclusions about the underlying anatomical structures (Mori &
Tournier, 2014).

Diffusion–weighted data is obtained by applying additional
diffusion-encoding gradients during an MRI scan. As explained
in Section 5.1.1, all protons resonate with the same frequency
in the homogenous B_0 field. Applying an in-homogenous,

diffusion-encoding gradient on top of the B_0 de-phases the protons. After the gradient is switched off again, the protons resonate at different frequencies depending on their position. To
obtain information about diffusion, a second gradient field with
the reversed polarity relative to the first one is applied. Due to
the reversed polarity, this field restores the phase of the protons.
Importantly, a complete re-phasing can only occur if no molecular motion occurs between the application of the diffusion-
encoding gradients. Protons that moved due to diffusion will
not be in phase with the other protons after use of the second
gradient. Hence, the signal will be lower compared to the signal
obtained before gradient application. Consequently, the extent of
signal loss contains information about the amount of diffusion
occurring, which in turn indicates the structure of the tissue un-
derneath (Mori & Tournier, 2014).

The signal loss measured due to proton movement can be
formulated with the following equation defined by Stejskal and
Tanner (1965):

$$\frac{S_g}{b_0} = e^{-bD(g)} \tag{5.3}$$

In Equation 5.3, g denotes the direction of the gradient, S_g
represents the strength of the signal, b_0 is an MRI-signal with
minimal diffusion weighting and the factor b is a constant determined by the parameters of the measurement. Importantly, $D(g)$
denotes the diffusion coefficient in the direction of the gradient
g which is to be determined from the other known parameters
and empirical data S_g.

5.4.1.1   *The diffusion tensor*

The amount and directionality of water motion as measured via dMRI is commonly visualised as geometrical shapes. Isotropic diffusion—i. e. random movement into any direction—is represented as a sphere (left side in Figure 5.5). As it uniformly extends into all directions, the radius of this sphere is sufficient to describe the directionality of diffusion. Therefore, in case of isotropic proton movement, the coefficient $D(g)$ alone indicates the strength of diffusion.

In contrast to this scalar value for the isotropic case, six values are required to describe an ellipsoid used to visualise anisotropic diffusion: the orientation of the three principle axes together with their lengths (right side in Figure 5.5). In order obtain these six values, a so-called diffusion tensor D is needed. This tensor is visualised as a 3×3 symmetrical matrix. As a minimal requirement, at least six diffusion-weighted volumes and one image without diffusion–weighting (i. e.the b_0 image) have to be recorded to obtain the six unknown values for this tensor.

Computing the three eigenvalues λ_1, λ_2 and λ_3 and the three eigenvectors v_1, v_2 and v_3 of the tensor matrix yields the missing parameters for the diffusion ellipsoid: the eigenvalues describe the lengths of the longest, middle and shortest perpendicular axes, while the eigenvectors describe their respective orientation. The eigenvalues serve as the basis to derive diffusion indices like fractional anisotropy (FA) and mean diffusivity (MD).

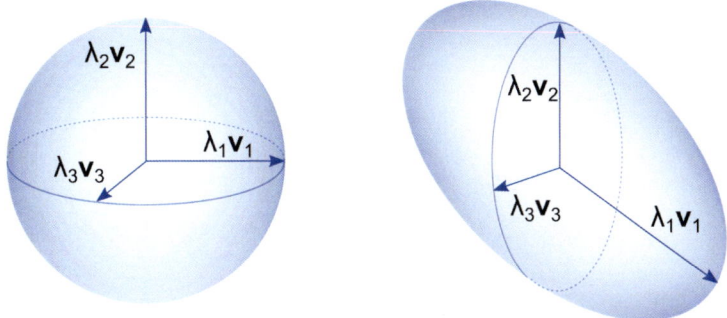

Figure 5.5: Geometrical visualisation of different diffusion properties. Left: isotropic diffusion represented by a sphere with $\lambda_1 = \lambda_2 = \lambda_3$. Right: anisotropic diffusion, represented by an ellipsoid with $\lambda_1 > \lambda_2 \geq \lambda_3$.

FRACTIONAL ANISOTROPY.   Differences between the three tensor eigenvalues λ_1, λ_2 and λ_3 determine the FA (Mori & Tournier, 2014):

$$FA = \sqrt{\frac{1}{2}} \frac{\sqrt{(\lambda_1 - \lambda_2)^2 + (\lambda_2 - \lambda_3)^2 + (\lambda_3 - \lambda_1)^2}}{\sqrt{\lambda_1^2 + \lambda_2^2 + \lambda_3^2}} \qquad (5.4)$$

Thus, FA indicates the extent of anisotropy. For isotropic diffusion with $\lambda_1 = \lambda_2 = \lambda_3$, the FA is 0. Higher FA values approaching one indicate a more elongated shape of the diffusion ellipsoid caused by more anisotropic proton movement.

MEAN DIFFUSIVITY.   MD is defined as the mean of the three eigenvalues λ_1, λ_2 and λ_3 (Mori & Tournier, 2014):

$$MD = \frac{\lambda_1 + \lambda_2 + \lambda_3}{3} \tag{5.5}$$

As follows, MD indicates the average amount of diffusion. Strong isotropic and strong anisotropic diffusion result in high MD.

Axonal diameter, fibre density and the degree of myelination all impact the directionality of diffusion and thus FA and MD (Mori & Tournier, 2014). Consequently, variations of tensor derived measures have been taken to indicate anatomical variability that is in turn associated with more efficient information processing in the brain (Kanai & Rees, 2011).

5.4.1.2   *Probabilistic tractography and streamline density*

Beyond measuring diffusion anisotropy within individual voxels, tractography techniques—most notably probabilistic tractography—provide functionality to re-construct white matter fibre pathways. Maps generated in this way are assumed to reflect whole collections of axons that establish structural connectivity between two regions (Mori & Tournier, 2014).

Tractography is based on the computation of a local diffusion model quantifying the principle fibre directions. Probabilistic models specifically estimate distributions of likely fibre directions within each voxel given the empirical data. In this

way, tracking based on so-called multi-fibre models is additionally sensitive to non-dominant fibre directions and can disentangle complex white matter configurations such as crossing fibres (Behrens, Johansen-Berg, Jbabdi, Rushworth, & Woolrich,
2007; Behrens et al., 2003). The ball-and-stick model used in the
current empirical studies is an example of such a multi-fibre
model, deriving several anisotropic 'sticks' that each represent
a distinct fibre orientation. During tracking, so-called streamlines are constructed by successively sampling from these distributions in a stepwise fashion. This process is started within
specified seed voxels and terminates when particular target voxels are reached. Importantly, streamlines that meet certain exclusion criteria (e.g.biologically unfeasible curvature) are dis-
carded from the final tractogram. As a result, volumetric maps
signifying the number of streamlines that were fit through each
voxel during tracking are generated, reflecting the connection
probability. Thus, analysis of streamline density maps provides
more comprehensive information about tract shape, and has
been shown to reflect connectivity more reliably than anisotropy
measures in terms of test-retest performance (Buchanan, Pernet,
Gorgolewski, Storkey, & Bastin, 2014).

5.5 EXAMINING FUNCTIONAL COHERENCE OF NEU-
RAL SYSTEMS

As explained in Section 5.2, MRI can be used to detect changes in
blood oxygenation across different brain areas. Importantly, the

brain exhibits systematic regional covariations even in absence of specific tasks, and this intrinsic activity shows patterns of remarkable temporal consistency across regions (Raichle, 2011). In their seminal study, Biswal, Zerrin Yetkin, Haughton, and Hyde (1995) reported systematic correlations between the low frequency domain of signals measured in areas associated with motor function at rest. Biswal et al. suggested these patterns to reflect the functional connectivity of the brain.

In the light of the current thesis investigating children as young as five years of age, rsfMRI offers several benefits. Its advantages include that no effortful task is needed for the participants to perform in the scanner. Furthermore, a single functional scan is sufficient to examine a range of different brain networks.

Approaches for analysing the brain's functional networks based on rsfMRI data include functional connectivity and coherence measures like regional homogeneity (ReHo) and fractional amplitude of low frequency fluctuations (fALFF).

5.5.1 *Resting state functional connectivity*

Resting state functional connectivity analyses provide the means to quantify the degree of synchronisation of spontaneous low-frequency fluctuations from rsfMRI data. Preprocessing includes motion correction and, optionally, techniques including the regression of average signals derived from the whole brain or individual tissue types out of each grey matter voxel's time series (Murphy & Fox, 2017; Muschelli et al., 2014). After low-pass filtering and smoothing, individual timecourses are correlated to compute the functional connectivity. This correlation may be carried out either in a voxel by voxel fashion, or—in terms of seed-based functional connectivity—based on mean timecourses of a priori defined ROIs. Positive correlations reflect functional coupling, while negative correlations have been suggested to differentiate contrasting neural processes or representations (see Figure 5.6; Fox, Snyder, Vincent, Corbetta, & Raichle, 2005).

Functional connectivity has been shown to covary with individual differences in behaviour across domains as variable as intelligence (Song et al., 2008), working memory (Hampson, Driesen, Roth, Gore, & Constable, 2010; Hampson, Driesen, Skudlarski, Gore, & Constable, 2006), and reading (M. Zhang et al., 2014). Additionally, Evans et al. (2015) demonstrated that rsfMRI functional connectivity between regions predicts long-term numerical abilities of children.

5.5.2 *Regional homogeneity*

ReHo represents a local functional measure that quantifies the coherence of timeseries within a confined neighbourhood of voxels (Zang, Jiang, Lu, He, & Tian, 2004). Specifically, it is defined as Kendall's coefficient concordance (Siegel, 1956) of a given voxel with the voxels within its immediate vicinity:

$$ReHo = \frac{\sum\limits_{i=0}^{n} (R_i)^2 - n(\overline{R})^2}{\frac{1}{12}K^2(n^3 - n)} \tag{5.6}$$

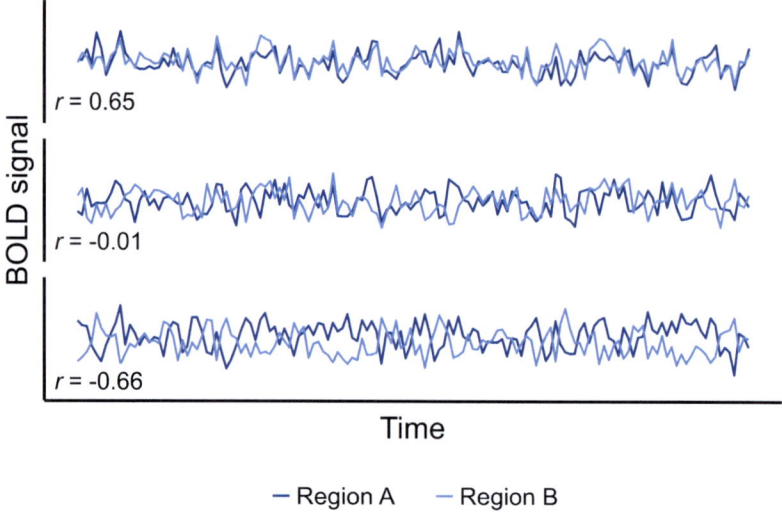

Figure 5.6: Schematic illustration of different synchronisation levels of spontaneous low-frequency fluctuations for two exemplary regions, based on simulated data. Top: Timecourses exhibiting a strong positive functional correlation, i. e. positive functional connectivity (r=0.65). Middle: Timecourses showing no correlation (r=-0.01). Bottom: Timecourses exhibiting a strong negative functional correlation, i. e.negative functional connectivity (r=-0.66).

where the sum rank for timepoint i is denoted by R_i; the average R_i for the number of ranks n is denoted by $\overline{R}$ and K denotes the size of the neighbourhood around the given voxel under consideration. The number of ranks n is typically defined to be 78. ReHo may range from zero to one, with higher values indicating that the timeseries of the examined neighbourhood of voxels is temporally more homogeneous. Advantages of this measure include its robustness against outliers and temporospatial noise, as well as its high test–retest reliability (Zuo et al., 2013).

This local similarity measure has been used to shed light onto the functional organisation of the prefrontal cortex and the ven-

tral visual stream (Jiang et al., 2015), predict individual performance in executive functioning (Tian, Ren, & Zang, 2012) and
distinguish typical from clinical samples suffering from neurodevelopmental disorders (Cao et al., 2006; Paakki et al., 2010).

5.5.3 *Fractional amplitude of low frequency fluctuations*

A further measure to examine the brain's intrinsic functional architecture is the fALFF. To obtain the fALFF for a given voxel,
the frequency spectrum of the pre-processed data is determined
first. Subsequently, the sum of amplitude across the whole frequency spectrum (i. e.0–0.25 Hz) along with the amplitude over
the low frequency range (i. e.0.01–0.08 Hz) are computed. fALFF
corresponds to the ratio of the low-frequency amplitude to the
amplitude to the whole range (Zou et al., 2008). Thus, this measure represents the relative contribution of the low frequency
oscillations to the entire frequency range. Importantly, it is relatively insensitive to physiological noise, especially near blood
vessels, cisterns and ventricles (Zuo et al., 2010).

Over the last decade, fALFF has been used increasingly to
identify alterations in the functional architecture of clinical populations (Egorova, Veldsman, Cumming, & Brodtmann, 2017;
Fryer et al., 2015; Hoptman et al., 2010). In healthy participants,
fALFF helped to identify functional plasticity in ageing populations following cognitive training (Yin et al., 2014). Developmen-
tally, it has been shown to vary across multiple brain regions in

children with low mathematical performance (Jolles, Supekar, et al., 2016).

5.6   STATISTICAL ANALYSIS

Given the various measures of brain structure and function described above, mainly two alternative approaches of statistical inference can be followed: whole-brain voxel-wise or ROI analyses, respectively.

To identify group-specific or behaviourally relevant variations on a whole-brain level, the respective maps of structural and functional measures are derived as explained above. Subsequently, fitting general linear models allows for a statistical analysis that takes pertinent covariates into account (Friston et al., 2007). Employing this kind of model, so-called statistical parametric maps are produced. These highlight areas of significant differences between groups or regions that correlate with performance after an appropriate correction for multiple comparisons has been performed (Mechelli et al., 2005).

As a more hypothesis driven approach, a ROI analysis offers an alternative to this voxel-wise examination of MRI data. Here, the search space for possible group differences or correlations with behaviour is focused on regions defined beforehand anatomically, functionally, or based on the available literature.

CHAPTER 6

EMPIRICAL STUDY I: UNRAVELING POTENTIAL CAUSES FROM CONSEQUENCES OF DEVELOPMENTAL DYSLEXIA

Empirical study I examines the neurobiological origins of developmental dyslexia (DD). To this end, it rests upon a longitudinal dataset of children that underwent psychometric testing and multimodal MRI before and after literacy instruction in school (i.e. at 5–6 years in kindergarten and 7–8 years in second grade).

6.1 INTRODUCTION

As explained in Section 2.1.2.1, DD is a heterogeneous condition: affected individuals show different cognitive deficits (Stefan Heim et al., 2008) and various theories of its neurobiological origin exist. However, formulated claims are primarily based on data of adult or school-aged participants. Therefore, they have to be regarded with caution, as observed differences between cases and controls might in fact be driven by a disparate amount and quality of literacy experience (see Section 2.1.2.2).

To date, only limited evidence of predisposing neurobiological factors distinguishing children with and without DD before literacy training is available. Longitudinal EEG studies suggest that future dyslexics show reduced electrophysiological responses to speech already 2–5 months after birth (Schaadt et al., 2015; van Zuijen, Plakas, Maassen, Maurits, & van der Leij, 2013). For instance, van Zuijen et al. demonstrated that the auditory system of infants who become non-fluent readers fails to discriminate between syllables with variable consonant onsets such as /bAk/ vs. /dAk/.

Moreover, evidence provided from a neuroimaging perspective suggests early anomalies with respect to structure and function of regions that will later become part of the dorsal reading network. Specifically, cortical thickness in left temporal and parietal cortices was shown to be reduced in future dyslexic children (Clark et al., 2014; Kraft et al., 2015), together with reduced myelination of the arcuate fasciculus, the white matter pathway connecting these areas with premotor and inferior frontal regions (Kraft et al., 2016).

Accordingly, the sparse data currently available indicated atypical functioning and maturation of an extended brain system supporting phonological processing. However, direct and consistent integration of these disjointed findings into a framework explaining the aetiology of DD is constrained by disparity of samples and methods in previous work. What is more, comprehensive research needs to also investigate the potential predisposing relevance of competing theories highlighting other sensory or cognitive domains (see Section 2.1.2.1).

The present study aims to systematically test whether existing neurobiological theories of DD reflect potential developmental causes rather than consequence. To this end, resting-state fMRI, T_1- and diffusion-weighted imaging data were acquired before and after literacy instruction in school. Combining these multimodal measures, we scrutinised the contribution of complex cortical and subcortical networks that were previously linked to the aetiology of DD (see Table 6.1). Importantly, we controlled statistical models for sociodemographic factors (maternal education), domain-general cognitive capacities (non-verbal IQ, attention) and comorbid learning disorders to reveal anomalies specific to the emergence of DD (see Sections 2.3 and 2.4).

6.2   METHODS

6.2.1   *Participants*

82 native German-speaking children were recruited from the Leipzig metropolitan area. The main target group of the recruitment procedure were individuals with at least one first-degree relative with DD in order to maximise the number of cases in the final sample. Accordingly, 37 of the 82 children had a familial risk of developing dyslexia. Written informed consent and verbal informed assent to participate were obtained from all parents and children, respectively. The study was approved by the Ethics Committee of the University of Leipzig, Germany, and followed American Psychological Association (APA) standards

Table 6.1: Cortical and subcortical networks that were previously linked to the aetiology of developmental dyslexia.

Assumed core deficit	Target regions	Target tracts
Phonological deficit	A1 (Lehongre et al., 2011)	A1 →PT
	PT (Lehongre et al., 2011)	PT →BA6
	BA6 (Dufor, Serniclaes, Sprenger-Charolles, & Démonet, 2009)	PT →BA44
	BA44 (Kraft et al., 2016)	
Sensory processing deficits		
visual system	LGN (Livingstone et al., 1991)	LGN →V1
	V1 (Livingstone et al., 1991)	LGN →MT
	MT (Eden et al., 1996)	V1 →VTOC
auditory system	IC (Hornickel & Kraus, 2013)	IC →MGB
	MGB (Galaburda et al., 1994)	MGB →A1
	A1 (Clark et al., 2014; Lehongre et al., 2011)	
orthographic system	VTOC (Salmelin, Service, Kiesilä, Uutela, & Salonen, 1996)	VTOC →PT
		VTOC →BA45/47
Cerebellar deficit	cerebellum (Nicolson et al., 1999)	

A1 = primary auditory cortex; PT = planum temporale; BA = Brodmann area; LGN = lateral geniculate nucleus; V1 = primary visual cortex; MT = middle temporal visual area; VTOC = ventral occipitotemporal cortex; IC = inferior colliculus; MGB = medial geniculate nucleus

in accordance with the declaration of Helsinki (World Medical Association, 2013).

Of the 82 initially recruited children, 39 individuals were excluded from further analyses because they *(i)* received a diagnosis of attention deficit hyperactivity disorder ($n = 4$, determined based on parental questionnaire), *(ii)* did not have complete structural MRI datasets (i.e., did not comply with the experimental procedures in a training session, exhibited excessive movement during the MRI scan or were unable to attend follow-up sessions, $n = 24$), *(iii)* did not finish all psychometric tests ($n = 7$) or *(iv)* performed below the 16th percentile in a standardised math test (to exclude cases of developmental dyscalculia, $n = 4$). One additional participant had to be excluded due to an experimental error during psychometric testing. In the remaining sample of 42 children, dyslexia was diagnosed based on standardised and age-normed reading and spelling tests. Performance below the 16th percentile rank of the population performance in at least one of the tests led to assignment to the dyslexic group. Correspondingly, individuals performing above the 25th percentile rank were assigned to the control group if they had neither first- nor second-degree relatives with developmental dyslexia. Applying these criteria, 16 children were classified as dyslexic and 16 children were classified as typically developing controls (Table 6.2). None of the participants in the final sample scored below 85 on average in the two non-verbal IQ tests. Note that additionally, two controls had to be excluded from rsfMRI analysis of kindergarten data, and two dyslexic cases were excluded from the functional data analysis of school-age data due to excessive head motion during the respective scans.

6.2.2   *Behavioral cognitive assessment and sociodemographic status*

All children underwent psychometric assessment at the two time points, that is, before they acquired literacy skills (age 5–6 in kindergarten) and again after first literacy instruction at the end of second grade (age 8–9; mean time between measurements: 2 years, 11 months; range of time between measurements: 2 years, 2 months – 3 years, 8 months). At kindergarten age, the following measures were derived:

Table 6.2: Overview of demographic information and psychometric performance of participants.

	Before literacy instruction				After literacy instruction			
	Dyslexia	Control	statistic	P value	Dyslexia	Control	statistic	P value
Demographic information								
N	16	16	...	...	16	16	...	...
Age[a]	5;8±4	5;6±4	U=169	0.139[b]	8;8±3	8;4±3	t(29)=-3.35	0.0022[c]
Sex (male / female)	11/5	9/7	odd's ratio=1.68	0.716[d]	...	...	...	...
Maternal education[e]	3.94±0.98	4.63±1.15	U=84	0.0893[b]	...	...	...	...
Handedness (laterality quotient)[e]	79.06±15.22	65.38±39.63	U=148.5	0.4344[b]	...	...	...	...
Familial risk status[f]	10/16	0/16	...	...	...	...	...	...
Psychometric assessment								
Non-verbal IQ[e]	99±12	109±12	t(29)=2.39	0.0236[c]	107±13	114±13	t(29)=1.66	0.1081[c]
Phonological short-term memory[e]	9±1.93	10.25±1.77	U=179.5	0.0473[b]	...	...	...	...
Phonological awareness[e]	32.16±4.72	35.38±3.59	t(29)=2.19	0.0368[c]	21.88±17.84	62.63±20.78	U=236	<0.0001[b]
Rapid automatised naming[e]	6.06±2.02	6.81±1.05	U=162	0.1790[b]	...	...	...	...
Spelling accuracy[e]	...	...	...	...	15.19±15.52	55.94±22.83	U=240	<0.0001[b]
Reading speed[e]	...	...	...	...	16.16±24.60	68.47±22.56	U=238	<0.0001[b]
Mathematical ability[e]	...	...	...	...	43.63±26.06	86.69±11.29	U=230	0.0001[b]

[a] years; months, age at MRI-scan, mean ± standard deviation in months
[b] Wilcoxon-Mann-Whitney U test (data not normally distributed)
[c] Welch two sample t-test (data normally distributed)
[d] Fisher's exact test
[e] mean ± standard deviation
[f] familial risk of DD / no familial risk of DD

HANDEDNESS.   Using an adapted version of the Edinburgh Handedness Inventory (Oldfield, 1971), we assessed children's handedness in terms of their laterality quotient (LQ), with scores ranging from -100 (left handed) to 100 (right handed). Left-handedness is defined as an LQ < -28, individuals with an LQ > 48 are considered to be right-handed, and ambidexterity is defined as values greater -28 and smaller than 48.

NON-VERBAL INTELLIGENCE.   Pre-school non-verbal intelligence was quantified using the performance IQ subscale of the Wechsler preschool and primary scale of intelligence (WPPSI-III; Wechsler, Petermann, & Lipsius, 2009). The average normed IQ score is 100 with a standard deviation of ± 15.

PHONOLOGICAL SHORT-TERM MEMORY.   Using the digit span subtest of the Kaufmann Assessment Battery for Children (K-ABC III; Kaufman, Kaufman, Melchers, & Preuß, 2009), we assessed children's preschool phonological short-term memory. In this test, number sequences of ascending length have to be recalled. The sequence span increases every three items from two to maximally nine until all three items of a length are reproduced incorrectly. Children receive a point for each correctly recalled number sequence.

PHONOLOGICAL AWARENESS (PA).   A composite measure from rhyming, sound association, syllable segmentation, and sound-to-word matching tasks from the Bielefeld screening of literacy precursor abilities (BISC; Jansen, Mannhaupt, Marx, & Skowronek, 1999) were computed as a measure of phonological awareness (PA). The final score corresponds to the combined number of correct responses in all subtests, with a maximal value of 40 (10 per task).

RAPID AUTOMATISED NAMING (RAN).   To test for children's ability to retrieve phonological representations, we used the rapid automatised naming (RAN) subtest of the BISC (Jansen et al., 1999). This task required children to rapidly name colours of 24 visually presented black and white objects while the time needed for completion was recorded. Raw values are converted into scores ranging from zero to eight.

MATERNAL EDUCATION.   As a measure of sociodemographic status, mothers were asked to fill out a self-constructed questionnaire assessing their highest school degree (4-point scale: no degree – o points; German 'Abitur' [high school diploma/A level] – 3 points) and vocational qualification (5-point scale: no qualification – o points; German 'Habilitation' [postdoctoral academic qualification] – 4 points). Overall maternal education score corresponds to sum of both subscales.

Testing at the end of second grade included the following measures:

NON-VERBAL INTELLIGENCE.   Using the perceptual reasoning IQ subscale of the Wechsler intelligence scale for children (WISC-IV; Petermann & Petermann, 2011), we assessed individual non-verbal intelligence at the end of second grade. The average normed IQ score is 100 with a standard deviation of $\pm$ 15.

PHONOLOGICAL AWARENESS.   The average standardised percentile ranks from pseudoword segmentation, vowel-replacement, word completion, phoneme exchange, sound categorization, vowel length judgment, and word reversal subtests of the Basic competences for reading and writing abilities test (BAKO; Stock, Marx, & Schneider, 2003) were used to assess children's PA at school age.

SPELLING ACCURACY.   Children were asked to write after dictation as part of an age-normed, standardised German spelling test (DERET1-2; Stock & Schneider, 2008). Percentile ranks based on the respective spelling accuracy were measured.

READING SPEED.   To assess reading speed, the corresponding percentile rank based on number of words a child correctly read within 1 minute as part of the Salzburg test of reading and spelling, second edition (SLRT-II; Moll & Landerl, 2010) was used.

MATHEMATICAL ABILITY.   Mathematical competence at the end of second grade in school was quantified using the Heidelberg computation test (HRT; Haffner, Baro, Parzer, & Resch, 2005) that comprises two subscales. The first quantifies early arithmetic abilities with subtests requiring basic addition and subtraction, solving simple equations and greater-or-smaller-than comparisons. The second subscale assesses visuospatial skills, providing a composite score of tasks that require children to estimate the length of line-drawings and the number of elements needed to build given block figures, to count shapes in a visual array, to connect spatially scrambled numerals in ascending order and to extract the logical rule determining the sequence of a particular row of numbers. General mathematical ability was defined as the composite score of both subscales.

6.2.3 *Magnetic resonance imaging data acquisition*

At kindergarten age, a training session using a mock scanner was conducted first to familiarise children with the MRI procedure and maximise compliance. In a next session, scanning was performed on a 3 T Siemens TIM Trio magnetic resonance scanner (Siemens AG, Erlangen, Germany) with a 12 channel radio-frequency head coil.

T_1-WEIGHTED IMAGING.   To obtain reliable T_1 maps, a magnetization-prepared 2 rapid acquisition gradient echo sequence (MP2RAGE, Marques et al., 2010) was acquired with the following parameters: repetition time of the total sequence cycle (TR) = 5000ms; first inversion time (TI_1) = 700ms; flipangle α_1 = 4°; second inversion time (TI_2) = 2500ms; flipangle α_2 = 5°; echo time (TE) = 2.82ms; field of view (FOV) = 250 × 219 × 188mm; voxel size = 1.3mm³; generalised auto-calibrating partially parallel acquisitions (GRAPPA) factor = 3.

DIFFUSION-WEIGHTED IMAGING. Diffusion-weighted data were acquired using the echo planer imaging (EPI) method (parameters: TE = 83 ms; TR = 8000 ms; voxel size = 1.86mm x 1.86mm x 1.90mm³; FOV = 186 × 186 × 126). Overall, two sets of diffusion-weighted measurements were obtained. The first set was acquired along the anterior-to-posterior phase-encoding direction with 60 diffusion-encoding gradient directions and a b-value of 1000 s/mm². Additionally, seven volumes without diffusion-weighting were obtained, one at the beginning and the remaining interleaved after each block of 10 diffusion-weighted images. The second set of diffusion measurements was acquired along the reverse, posterior-to-anterior phase-encoding direction, consisting of one volume without and one with diffusion-weighting (b-value = 1000 s/mm²). Both sets are used to correct for artifacts such deformations induced by magnetic field inhomogeneities later in the analysis.

RESTING-STATE FMRI. Resting-state fMRI data was acquired on the same system using a T_{2^*} gradient-echo echo-planar imaging (EPI) sequence with the following parameters:

TR = 2000 ms; TE = 30 ms; flip angle α = 90°; FOV = 192 × 192 × 111 mm; 28 slices; resolution: 3.00 × 3.00 × 3.99 mm³; 100 volumes.

A second MRI session was performed when children were at the end of second grade on the same scanner upgraded to a 3T Prisma system, using a 64 channel head coil.

T_1-WEIGHTED IMAGING. T_1 maps were acquired using an MP2RAGE sequence with parameters TR = 5000ms; TI_1 = 700ms; flipangle α_1 = 4°; TI_2 = 2500ms; flipangle α_2 = 5°; TE = 2.01ms; FOV = 256 × 240 × 176mm; voxel size = 1.0mm3; GRAPPA factor = 2).

DIFFUSION-WEIGHTED IMAGING.   Comparable to the measurement at kindergarten age, two sets of diffusion-weighted imaging data were acquired using the EPI method (parameters: TE = 73 ms; TR = 4700 s; voxel size = 1.72 × 1.72 × 1.70 mm; FOV = 210 × 204 × 133). Again, in the first set of measurements, acquisition was along the anterior-to-posterior phase-encoding direction with 60 diffusion-encoding gradient directions and a b-value of 1000 s/mm². Additionally, eight volumes without diffusion-weighting were obtained, two at the beginning and the remaining interleaved after each block of 10 diffusion-weighted volumes. The second set of diffusion measurements was acquired along the reverse, posterior-to-anterior phase-encoding direction, consisting of one image without and one image with diffusion-weighting (b-value = 1000 s/mm^2) as a basis for later correction for inhomogeneity induced deformations.

RESTING-STATE FMRI.   150 volumes of rsfMRI data were acquired on the updated system with an EPI sequence with parameters TR = 2000 ms; TE = 30 ms; flip angle α = 90°; FOV = 192 × 192 × 127 mm; 32 slices; resolution: 3.00 × 3.00 × 3.99 mm^3.

6.2.4 *Magnetic resonance imaging data preprocessing*

T1-WEIGHTED IMAGES.   Initial preprocessing of T$_1$ brain images was performed using Version 5.3.0 of the FreeSurfer image analysis suite (Fischl, 2012; FreeSurfer, 2014). Thereby, data were motion corrected (Reuter & Fischl, 2011) and brain tissue was extracted using a hybrid watershed/surface deformation procedure (Ségonne et al., 2004).

These extracted brain images were subsequently rigidly aligned to an unbiased, asymmetric template for paediatric data in Montreal Neurological Institute (MNI) standard space, derived from 82 children aged 4.5–8.5 years (Fonov et al., 2011; Fonov et al., 2009). Common group templates were created from the individual T$_1$ images in MNI space for each of the two timepoints using Version 2.2.0 of the Advanced Normalization Tools (ANTs; Avants, Tustison, & Johnson, 2017; Avants et al., 2011; Avants et al., 2010), adapted for paediatric data as in Cafiero, Brauer, Anwander, and Friederici (2018).

DIFFUSION-WEIGHTED DATA.   Prior   to   preprocessing,
dMRI data was screened for motion artifacts by a semi-
automatic method identifying intensity dropouts in the diffusion signal caused by motion (Schreiber, Riffert, Anwander, &
Knösche, 2014). Additionally, directions were visually inspected
for artifacts (Soares, Marques, Alves, & Sousa, 2013; Tournier,
Mori, & Leemans, 2011). Preprocessing of dMRI data was performed the FMRIB Software Library (FSL, Version 5.0.9; FMRIB
Analysis Group, 2015; Jenkinson, Beckmann, Behrens, Woolrich,
& Smith, 2012).

In order to correct for motion, diffusion volumes were rigidly
aligned to the first b_0 image (Jenkinson, Bannister, Brady, &
Smith, 2002; Jenkinson & Smith, 2001). To compensate for inhomogeneity induced deformations, the susceptibility-induced off-
resonance field was computed based on the diffusion-weighted
image pairs acquired with opposite polarity of phase-encoding
(FSL's TOPUP; Andersson, Skare, & Ashburner, 2003; S. M.
Smith et al., 2004). Additionally, dMRI data were rigidly aligned
to the T_1-weighted image in MNI standard space and interpo-
lated to 1mm voxel size. To preserve high data quality, all trans-
formations necessary for image correction and registration to
the individual T_1 anatomy in MNI space were combined and
applied in a single step of interpolation. The diffusion tensor
was estimated using FSL's DTIFIT. Finally, the fibre orientation
distribution for each voxel was determined using crossing fibre
bayesian estimation of diffusion parameters as implemented in
FSL (Behrens et al., 2003).

RESTING-STATE FMRI DATA.   Processing of rsfMRI data was
performed using FSL, MATLAB Version R2017b (The Math-
Works, Inc., 2017) and the Analysis of Functional NeuroImages
software (AFNI) Version 17.2.17 (Cox, 1996; Cox & Hyde, 1997;
Scientific and Statistical Computing Core, 2017). Preprocessing
included removal of the first four images of each scan to allow
for stabilization of magnetization followed by slice time correction. Volume-by-volume head motion was quantified by frame-
wise displacement (FD), defined as the sum of rotational and
translational rigid body realignment parameters from one volume to the next (J. D. Power, Barnes, Snyder, Schlaggar, & Petersen, 2012). Volumes with FD > 0.5mm were excluded from
further analysis. Following this criterion, the 75 or 100 volumes
with lowest FD values were retained for the two measurement
time points, respectively, to ensure an equal amount of data
per participant to be used in the analysis. Next, rsfMRI data
was masked to exclude non-brain voxels. To generate partial
volume maps for GM, WM and CSF, T_1 images in MNI space
were segmented (Y. Zhang, Brady, & Smith, 2001). WM and
CSF masks were first thresholded at 80% tissue probability, min-
imising partial voluming with grey matter, and then rigidly
aligned to rsfMRI space. We applied the anatomical CompCor
method (Behzadi, Restom, Liau, & Liu, 2007) in order to remove
scanner-related and physiological noise from the data, thereby
also attenuating persistent effects of motion (Muschelli et al.,
2014). Five principal components from WM and CSF were estimated on the rsfMRI data and regressed out together with

the six linearly detrended motion parameters previously determined. Unlike standard global signal regression approaches, this technique also uncovers anticorrelations between resting state networks (Chai, Castañón, Öngür, & Whitfield-Gabrieli, 2012), while avoiding spurious negative correlations (Murphy, Birn, Handwerker, Jones, & Bandettini, 2009). As a final step, the residual data was bandpass filtered at 0.01–0.1Hz and spatially smoothed with a 6mm FWHM kernel.

6.2.5   Voxel–based and surface–based morphometry

Further pre-processing of T_1 data were performed using the Computational Anatomy Toolbox (CAT12; Version r1109; Gaser & Dahnke, 2017) for SPM12 Update Revision Number 6906 (Friston et al., 2007; SPM12, 2016) in MATLAB Version R2017b (The MathWorks, Inc., 2017). T_1 data in template space were segmented into grey and white matter. For segmentation, SPM relies on anatomical priors provided as tissue probability maps. Since the tissue priors provided as a standard are obtained from adult data, we replaced them with custom tissue probability maps, derived from the common group template of the respective timepoint to account for the anatomical details of our developmental sample. Probabilistic maps of the individual tissue types were created using FSL's FAST (Y. Zhang et al., 2001). Tissue probabilities were normalised to sum to one. Finally, all maps were resampled to a voxel size of 1.5 mm^3 and smoothed using a 35mm FWHM kernel, to approximate the resolution and smoothness of SPM's default anatomical priors. Additionally, grey and white matter maps created this way also replaced the default template for the fast diffeomorphic image registration procedure (DARTEL; Ashburner, 2007). Consequently, maps of grey matter volume (GMV), cortical thickness (CT), gyrification index (GI; Lüders et al., 2006), cortical folding complexity (CF; Yotter, Nenadic, et al., 2011) and sulcus depth (SD) were extracted for each participant. Finally, GMV data were smoothed using an 8 mm full width at half maximum (FWHM) kernel, while 15 mm kernels were used to smooth surface-based data.

6.2.6 *Regions of interest selection*

Participant-specific ROI masks (see Table 6.1) were obtained by aligning a multi-modal parcellation of brain areas comprising 180 cortical regions per hemisphere (Glasser et al., 2016, retrieved from https://balsa.wustl.edu/study/show/RVVG) to each participant's MNI-T_1 image for GMV, and to Freesurfer's fsaverage subject for CT, GI, CF, SD. The definition of ROIs in terms of regions defined in the multi-modal parcellation is given in Table 6.3.

Subcortical areas MGB, LGN, and the inferior colliculus (IC) were manually defined by two independent observers (the author of this thesis and Dr Michael A. Skeide) on a T_1 template with a resolution of 0.5mm^3 isotropic (Tardif et al., 2016). The overlap of both definitions was taken as final ROI. Location of thalamic regions corresponds to coordinates specified in the

Table 6.3: Definition of regions of interest in terms of regions defined in the multi-modal parcellation atlas (Glasser et al., 2016).

Region of interest	Atlas labels
left primary visual cortex (V1)	L_V1_ROI, 1
left middle temporal area (MT)	L_MT_ROI, 23
left fusiform gyrus (FG)	L_VVC_ROI, 163
left primary auditory cortex (A1)	L_A1_ROI, 24
,left planum temporale (PT)	L_LBelt_ROI, 174; L_PBelt_ROI, 124
left ventral premotor cortex (BA6)	L_6v_ROI, 56; L_6r_ROI, 78
left pars opercularis of the inferior frontal gyrus,(BA44)	L_44_ROI, 74
left pars triangularis/orbitalis of the inferior,frontal gyrus (BA45/47)	L_45_ROI, 75; L_47_ROI, 76

V1 = primary visual cortex; BA=Brodmann area; MT = middle temporal area; FG = fusiform gyrus; A1 = primary auditory cortex; PT = planun temporale; BA = Brodmann area; if several areas are given, they were combined to form the final ROI.

literature from other manual and connectivity-based segmentations (Devlin et al., 2006). Finally, the Spatially Unbiased Atlas Template (SUIT; Diedrichsen, 2006; Diedrichsen, Balsters, Flavell, Cussans, & Ramnani, 2009) of the cerebellum and brainstem were used to extract a cerebellar ROI.

6.2.7 *Tractography*

Structural connectivity was quantified by probabilistic tractography using probabilistic tractography as implemented in FM-RIB's Diffusion Toolbox as part of FSL (Behrens et al., 2007; Behrens et al., 2003). Each tract was generated by using each ROI involved once as seed and once as target for tracking. For each voxel in the grey/white matter interface region of the seed at hand, 5000 streamlines were initiated. Tracking was constrained by a curvature threshold of 0.2 and step length of 0.5 mm. Additionally, to quantify connectivity of the left planum temporale with inferior frontal regions BA6 and BA44 via the dorsal route only, we restricted tracking for the respective seed target pairs with a rectangular ventral exclusion mask. Likewise, tracking was restricted by both the ventral and an additional dorsal exclusion mask to quantify only local connectivity between the left primary auditory cortex and left planum temporale (see Figure 6.1). Specifically, the respective masks were defined within the commonMNI group templates for the respective time points. Position in y-direction of the ventral exclusion mask was 5mm anterior of the maximal y-coordinate of all subject's planum temporale seeds, spanning 3mm into the anterior direction (i.e. $y = 7 - 9$). In x- and z-direction, the plane extended from coordinare 0 into the negative directions (i.e. $x = 0 - -61$, $z = 0 - -49$), covering the entire anterior temporal lobe. The dorsal exclusion mask was defined as a plane covering the whole field of view in x- and y-direction for $z = 22 - 24$.

The resulting streamline density maps were first log-transformed and then divided in a voxel-wise manner by the log-transformed maximal number of possible streamlines. These log-transformed and normalised data were added for each tract. In order to obtain a mask for statistical analysis, individual participants' maps of combined connectivity indices were averaged and thresholded with the 80th percentile to extract only the core of the respective tract.

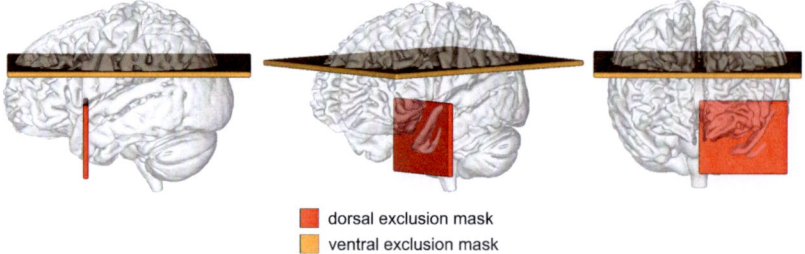

dorsal exclusion mask
ventral exclusion mask

Figure 6.1: Dorsal and ventral exclusion masks used to restrict tracking between planum temporale and frontal regions (red) and between primary auditory cortex and planum temporale (red and orange combined). Masks are displayed on a 3D rendering of the group template generated from subject's T_1 data acquired at the end of second grade.

6.2.8 Functional coherence measures

In order to investigate the local as well as the global similarity of time-series, we extracted regional homogeneity (ReHo; Zang et al., 2004, see Section 5.5.2) for a neighbourhood of $K=27$ voxels (see Section 5.5.2 and Equation 5.6). Additionally, we computed the fractional amplitude of low frequency fluctuations (fALFF; Zou et al., 2008, see Section 5.5.3), using the Data Processing Assistant for Resting-State fMRI toolbox (DPARSF; Yan & Zang, 2010), and finally converted into z-scores.

6.2.9 Statistical analysis

Demographic and behavioural data were tested for normality of distributions using the Shapiro-Wilk test. To compare groups, we used the non-parametric Wilcoxon-Mann-Whitney U test in case of non-normality, the Fisher's exact test for nominal data, and the Welch two sample t-test otherwise (all two-tailed).

ROI means of CT, CF, GI, SD, ReHo, fALFF, volumes of LGN, MGB, IC, and mean GMV of the cerebellum were extracted in MNI space. Mean functional connectivity was computed by extracting mean haemodynamic time-series for each ROI and calculating pair-wise correlations. FA and MD (see Section 5.4.1.1), as well as streamline density (see Section 5.4.1.2) were computed voxel-wise along the tracts identified by probabilistic tractography in SPM. ROI-wise or ROI-pair-wise comparisons of the different mean brain measures were performed using R–3.3.3 (R Core Team, 2016) by running multiple one-way analyses of covariance with covariates age, sex, handedness, maternal education, and arithmetic ability. Additionally, we included IQ acquired at the second timepoint as covariate for all analysis, because IQ measures were shown to be more reliable in school-age than in preschool children (Bishop et al., 2003).

Possible interactions between individual covariates and the categorical predictor variable were assessed beforehand to ensure homogeneity of regression slopes. A significant interaction was found between group and sex for functional connectivity between the left primary auditory cortex and the left planum temporale at kindergarten age. Consequently, separate analyses were run for male and female participants with respect to this comparison. No other significant interaction was found, indicating homogeneity of remaining regression curves. Within each comparison, results were family-wise-error corrected for number of ROIs. To test for potential effects not covered by our ROIs, we performed whole-brain analyses of each brain measure.

To assess prospective case-control discrimination based on neural and behavioural predictors, we calculated receiver operating characteristic curves. Variance inflation factor computed on all models indicated only weak multicollinearity between predictors (range 1.00-3.41). Areas under the receiver operating characteristic curve (AUC) of all models were compared using a two-tailed bootstrapping approach.

6.3   RESULTS

In terms of phonological short-term memory and phonological awareness, children with developmental dyslexia performed significantly worse compared to controls, both before literacy instruction at mean age 5y$\pm$7m (phonological short-term memory: $N = 32$, $U = 179.5$, p $= 0.0473$, d $= 0.75$, two-tailed; phonological awareness: $N = 32$, $t(28) = 2.19$, $p = 0.0368$, $d = 0.78$, two-tailed) and after literacy instruction at mean age 8y$\pm$6m (phonological awareness: $N = 32$, $U = 236$, $p < 0.0001$, $d = 2.06$, two-tailed; see Table 6.2). Furthermore, reading speed ($N = 32$, $U = 238$, $p < 0.0001$, $d = 2.14$, two-tailed) as well as spelling accuracy ($N = 32$, $U = 240$, $p < 0.0001$, $d = 2.23$, two-tailed) were significantly reduced in dyslexic cases versus controls.

Group comparisons of the various cortical and subcortical measures (see Figure 6.2) revealed a significant gyrification difference in terms of higher absolute mean curvature of the left primary auditory cortex in dyslexic children compared to controls, persistent across time points (before literacy: $N = 32$, $F(1,24) =$

9.64, $p = 0.0048$, $\eta^2 = 0.19$; after literacy: $N = 32$, $F(1,24) = 9.21$, $p = 0.0057$, $\eta^2 = 0.22$). Additionally, functional connectivity between left primary auditory cortex and left planum temporale was significantly lower in dyslexic children before literacy acquisition ($N = 30$, $F(1,24) = 14.73$, $p = 0.0009$, $\eta^2 = 0.32$). This effect was driven by a significant difference in boys ($N = 20$, $F(1,13) = 34.58$, $p = 0.0001$, $\eta^2 = 0.45$), but not girls ($N = 10$, $F(1,3) = 0.05$, $p = 0.8388$, $\eta^2 = 0.01$; see Figure 6.2).

In terms of white matter structural connectivity, we found significantly higher streamline density within the left arcuate fasciculus ($N = 32$, 70 voxels, $F(1,24) = 19.80$, $p = 0.004$, $\eta^2 = 0.45$), connecting the left planum temporale with the left ventral premotor area (BA 6). No other region-of-interest or whole-brain control analysis revealed any additional statistically significant effects for any measure under investigation.

Finally, to assess prospective case-control discrimination of the cortical differences identified in our analysis, predictive sensitivity and specificity of three models were compared: *(i)* a model comprising only the three significant neural indices, *(ii)* a model comprising the three most powerful behavioural predictors known from the literature (rapid automatised naming, phonological short-term memory, and phonological awareness; Moll, Ramus, et al., 2014; Raschle, Chang, & Gaab, 2011; Saygin et al., 2013; Ziegler et al., 2010), and *(iii)* a model combining both brain and behaviour. Data of 30 children with complete behavioural, structural and functional datasets at kindergarten age were used for model estimation. The area under the

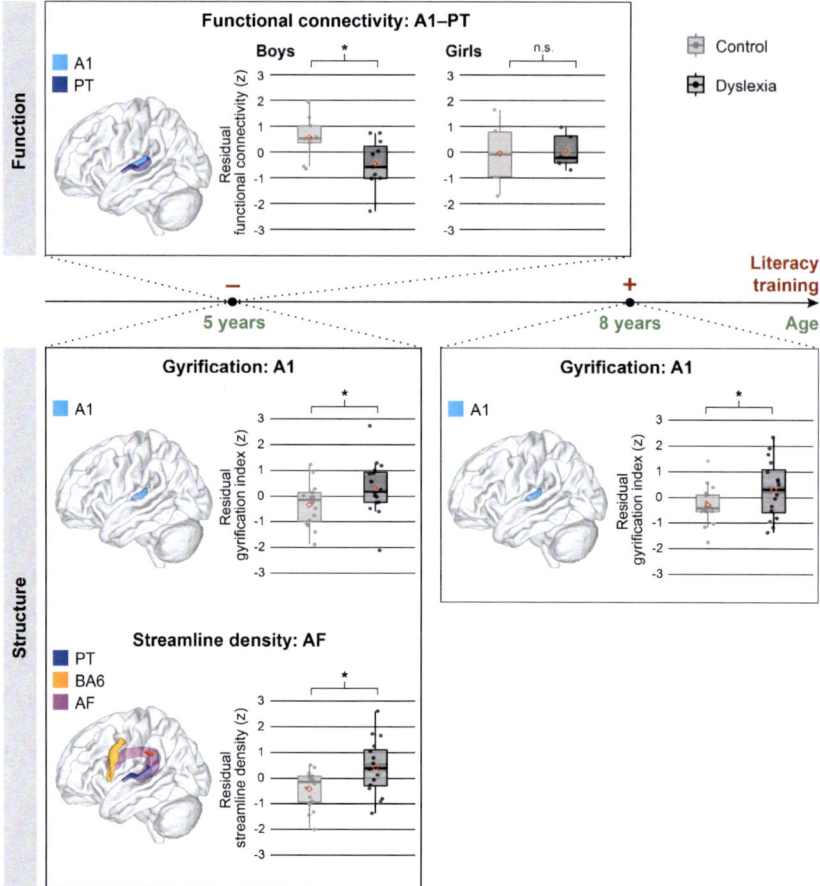

Figure 6.2: Overview of significant neural differences between dyslexic and control children. Horizontal lines within the box plots represent the group median. Vertical lines at the top and the bottom of the box plots depict the standard deviation. Red diamonds denote the mean of the distribution. Grey and black dots are individual data points. $N = 32$ for comparisons of structural measures, $N = 30$ for comparisons of functional connectivity. Asterisks indicate family-wise-error corrected differences significant at $p < 0.05$. A1 = primary auditory cortex; PT = planum temporale; BA6 = Brodmann area 6; AF = arcuate fasciculus.

receiver operating characteristic curve (AUC) of the first model was 0.86 (standard error (SE) = 0.07, 95% confidence interval (CI) = 0.72–1.00, $d = 1.53$). The AUC of the model based purely on behaviour was 0.76 (SE = 0.09, 95% CI = 0.58–0.94, d = 1.00), and the AUC of the combined model was 0.91 (SE = 0.05, 95% CI = 0.81–1.00, d = 1.90). Statistical comparison of AUCs showed that the combined model has significantly higher discrimination power than the purely behavioural model (D = -2.00, p = 0.0464), while there were no significant differences between AUCs of the neural model and the behavioural model (D = -0.95, p = 0.3429, two-tailed) and the combined model and the neural model (D = -0.91, p = 0.3644, two-tailed; see Figure 6.3).

6.4   DISCUSSION

In the present study, we aimed to distentangle potential causes of DD from the consequence of impoverished reading experience. All analyses relied on a longitudinal dataset that combines psychometric testing with brain measures derived from dMRI, T_1 and rsfMRI acquired before and after literacy instruction in school. Thereby, contributions of complex cortical and subcortical networks that were previously linked to the aetiology of reading and writing impairments were investigated systematically. Importantly, we took particular care to exclude cases of attention deficit hyperactivity disorder and developmental dyscalculia to reduce the potentially confounding role of prominent comorbidities of DD. Additionally, all analyses were carefully controlled for individual performance in mathematics such that reported findings reflect differences specifically related to literacy impairment.

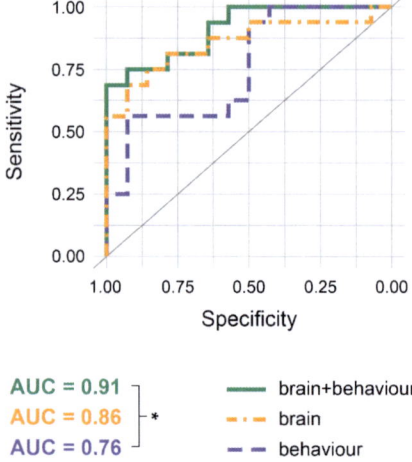

AUC = 0.91 ┐   ——— brain+behaviour
AUC = 0.86 ├ *   – · – brain
AUC = 0.76 ┘   – – behaviour

Figure 6.3: Receiver operating characteristic curves of models predicting later literacy outcome. Dashed/purple = model based
on behavioural measurements only, dotted-dashed/orange
= model based on neural indices identified in the current
study, solid/green = model based on combined neural
and behavioural measures, AUC = area under receiver operating characteristic curve. All measures were collected
prior to literacy training. Included behavioural measures
("behaviour") were phonological awareness, phonological
short-term memory, and rapid automatised naming. Included brain measures ("brain") comprised gyrification of
left primary auditory cortex, functional connectivity between left primary auditory cortex and planum temporale,
and streamline density of a cluster in the arcuate fasciculus.
The label "brain+behaviour" denotes a model combining
both behavioural and brain measures. $N = 30$ for all models. Asterisks indicate differences significant at $p < 0.05$
(two-tailed).

Our results show that pre-literate children who will face literacy deficits later in life have reduced phonological processing
skills compared to typically developing controls. Additionally,
we found altered gyrification patterns of the left primary auditory cortex and structural differences in terms of increased connectivity strength of the left arcuate fasciculus. Finally, dyslexic
boys—but not girls—exhibited decreased functional connectivity between the left primary auditory cortex and the planum

temporale. Preceding literacy acquisition, these effects point to predispositions rather than manifestations of DD. Moreover, due to our rigorous statistical control, they can also not be explained by individual differences in sociodemographic status, non-verbal IQ, attention or mathematical deficits. Interestingly, investigation of the same cohort at the end of second grade in school revealed only the difference in gyrification pattern of the left primary auditory cortex as a persistent anomaly in the dyslexic subgroup.

Behaviourally, phonological awareness, phonological short-term memory, and rapid automatised naming are consistently reported to be the most reliable predictors of reading attainment (Moll, Ramus, et al., 2014; Raschle et al., 2011; Saygin et al., 2013; Ziegler et al., 2010). In line with these reports, future dyslexic children and controls in the current study differed significantly in terms of phonological processing skills. In accord with this behavioural profile, we found cortical malformation and aberrant connectivity within these individuals, affecting a coherent network of brain areas known to specifically support speech sound processing (**Hypothesis I.a**).

In the first longitudinal MRI study investigating neural precursors of DD, Clark et al. (2014) also identified malformations of the left primary auditory cortex as the distinguishing feature between dyslexic cases and controls both before and after literacy instruction in school. In contrast to this earlier finding that focused on cortical thickness, however, our results highlight auditory cortex differences in terms of gyrification patterns, in line with postmortem work on adult dyslexics reporting polymicro-gyria (Galaburda et al., 2006, **Hypothesis I.b**). The reasons for this disparity are unclear. As the brain's folding patterns might be intrinsically linked to differential trajectories of cortical ex-pansion (Budday et al., 2014; Tallinen et al., 2016), it is possible that both studies capture a similar anomaly using different mea-sures. This is unlikely, however, as we provide a complementary analysis of cortical thickness that fails to replicate the previously reported differences. Additionally, since the analysis reported by Clark et al. (2014) was restricted to one measure, it is impossible to say whether the observed effects also co-occured with differ-ences in gyrification. Moreover, the work by Clark et al. (2014) has been criticised for its limited sample size (Kraft et al., 2015; Ramus et al., 2018) of comparing 7 dyslexic individuals with 10 controls before reading acquisition.

Remarkably, increased gyrification stood out as the sole signif-icantly different macroanatomical measure in our study, while cortical folding and thickness, as well as sulcus depth, were comparable between groups. In seminal histological work, Gal-aburda et al. (1985) identified a disproportionate number of small foldings, so-called polymicrogyria, in perisylvian cortical areas of dyslexic specimens. It seems possible that our gyrifica-tion measure may capture consequences of these anomalies. In fact, changes in cortical folding patterns rapidly decrease after birth (Li et al., 2014; T. White, Su, Schmidt, Kao, & Sapiro, 2010) and are thus often taken as a sensitive marker for deviant pre- and perinatal neuronal development (Bayly et al., 2014; Mutlu et al., 2013). Accordingly, the differences in gyrification reported here might best be explained in terms of prenatal genetic effects that disrupt formation of the auditory cortex, consequently leading to the phonological processing deficits frequently associated with literacy impairments. In fact, prominent candidate dyslexia genes have been linked to neuronal migration and axon guidance (R. L. Peterson & Pennington, 2012). Remarkably, one of the best characterised gene variants was shown to increase variability of neural responses in the primary auditory cortex of rodents, thereby hampering encoding of speech sounds (Centanni, Booker, et al., 2014; Centanni, Chen, et al., 2014).

With respect to functional coherence of the cortical and subcortical networks investigated, our finding of reduced functional connectivity between the left primary auditory cortex and planum temporale corroborates the large body of literature demonstrating the vital role of these areas for spectro-temporal analysis of the continuous speech stream (Giraud & Poeppel, 2012; Lehongre et al., 2011). Interestingly, our analysis revealed this effect to be driven by a significant difference in boys, but not in girls, thus confirming the functional aspect of **Hypothesis I.c** only for a specific subset of our study sample. Given the small sample sizes of the two gender subgroups, these results should be interpreted with caution. Still, it is noteworthy that typically more boys than girls show literacy deficits (Moll, Kunze, et al., 2014). Considering that we also replicated this gender imbalance in our study group, a possible hypothesis that warrants further investigation may be that deficits in functional coherence are less likely to occur in female than in male dyslexics.

Farther downstream, we found significantly increased stream-line density in a branch of the left arcuate fasciculus, connecting the planum temporale with the ventral premotor cortex (**Hypothesis I.c**). This finding is consistent with studies linking literacy and the structure of this tract (de Schotten et al., 2014; Yeatman et al., 2012). Moreover, it also accords with the long-standing view that children with literacy deficits increasingly rely on articulatory recoding strategies supported by the ventral premotor cortex to compensate for faulty speech encoding in the planum temporale (Pugh et al., 2000; Richlan, Kronbichler, & Wimmer, 2011; S. E. Shaywitz et al., 1998).

It is important to note that anomalous gyrification patterns were the only persistent neural difference observed both at pre-literate and school age. There are several possible reasons for the discontinuity of the functional and structural connectivity effects. One plausible—though speculative—explanation lies in distinct early maturational trajectories that fail to reach significance in later years (Yeatman et al., 2012). In fact, a similar observation was made by Yeatman et al. (2012), who demonstrated higher initial structure of the arcuate fasciculus in children with poor literacy abilities. What is more, in poor readers investigated cross-sectionally, FA subsequently declined until adolescence. Typically developing controls, in contrast, exhibited a continuous increase in FA during the same period.

Finally, a prospective classification model combining known behavioural predictors and the neural indices identified in our experiments proved excellent, above-chance discriminatory power with an area under the receiver operator characteristic curve (AUC) of 0.91. In contrast, prediction based on the behavioural performance alone did not distinguish between future dyslexics and controls. Importantly, a neural-only model derived from our significant MRI measures performed significantly above chance.

In conclusion, the results of empirical study I critically add to the understanding of neural underpinnings of DD. Specifically, we provide converging behavioural and neuroimaging evidence for a phonological deficit that manifests early in dyslexic individuals, even before literacy instruction has begun.

CHAPTER 7

EMPIRICAL STUDY II: SURFACE PLASTICITY AND NUMERACY SKILLS

Empirical Study II examines neural correlates of individual differences in typical mathematical ability. By providing an in-depth analysis of longitudinal changes of cortical surface anatomy during the first two years of school in typically developing children, I demonstrate how early cortical surface plasticity relates to basic numeracy skills.

7.1 INTRODUCTION

While a considerable amount of literature identifies the importance of specific brain areas for numerical-mathematical processing in adults (also see Section 2.2.1; Ansari et al., 2006; Knops et al., 2009; Menon, 2010; Piazza et al., 2004; Piazza et al., 2006; Piazza et al., 2007; Qin et al., 2014; Venkatraman et al., 2005), dynamic brain changes related to the acquisition of numeracy competence early in life is less well understood. Most developmental studies investigate mathematical development at school age (Evans et al., 2015; Qin et al., 2014; Rivera et al., 2005). In a seminal study, Cantlon et al. (2006) link specific brain areas have been linked to magnitude processing at a preschool age (Cantlon et al., 2006).

However, little is known about specific plastic changes of cortical surface anatomy relating to early mathematical performance in children at the transition from kindergarten to second grade. This initial period of first formal mathematical instruction is a crucial time for individual numeracy development, accompanied by a shift from counting-based to fact-retrieval strategies used for problem-solving as children master basic mathematical concepts (Cho et al., 2011). Therefore, the present study aims to characterise specific associations between components of early numeracy skills assessed in second grade of school and neuroplastic changes between five and eight years of age. Importantly, all analysis accounted for important confounds such as literacy skills and sociodemographic status.

7.2   METHODS

7.2.1   *Participants*

Participants of this study were selected from the same group of 82 inititially recruited children described in Chapter 6. Importantly, the focus of the second study presented in this thesis was on the association between cortical surface plasticity and early mathematical ability in typically developing individuals, rather than investigating neural correlates related to specific learning disorders. Therefore, different exclusion criteria from those used in the first empirical study applied. Consequently, data from a subset of 28 children of the initially recruited sample went into the current analysis (15 female; age range at kindergarten: 5 years, 0 months – 6 years, 0 months; mean ± SD: 5 years, 6 months ± 6 months; age range at second grade in school: 7 years, 11 months – 8 years, 11 months; mean ± SD: 8 years, 5 months ± 5 months). The remaining 54 children were excluded from further analysis because they received a diagnosis of attention deficit hyperactivity disorder ($n = 4$) or developmental dyslexia ($n = 9$, both determined based on a parental questionnaire), did not have complete datasets (i. e., did not comply with the experimental procedures in a training session, exhibited excessive movement during the MRI scan or were unable to attend follow-up sessions, $n = 22$), did not complete all psychometric measurements ($n = 3$), scored below the 20th percentile rank of the population performance in standardised and age-normed reading or spelling tests ($n = 12$) or performed below the 20th percentile in a standardised math test (clinical cases of developmental dyscalculia, $n = 3$). One other child had to be excluded due to an experimental error during psychometric testing. None of the remaining children scored below 85 on average in two non-verbal IQ tests.

7.2.2 *Behavioral cognitive assessment and sociodemographic status*

Assessment of psychometric measures and sociodemographic status has been described in Section 6.2.2.

7.2.3 *Magnetic resonance imaging data acquisition*

Details on MRI data acquisition have been described in Section 6.2.3. Note that only the T_1-weighted data were used in the current study.

7.2.4 *Magnetic resonance imaging data preprocessing*

Using Version 5.3.0 of the FreeSurfer image analysis suite (Fischl, 2012; FreeSurfer, 2014), T_1 brain images were corrected for motion (Reuter & Fischl, 2011). Brain tissue was extracted based on a hybrid watershed/surface deformation procedure (Ségonne et al., 2004) and rigidly aligned to an unbiased, asymmetric template for paediatric data in MNI standard space, derived from 82 children aged 4.5–8.5 years (Fonov et al., 2011; Fonov et al., 2009).

A common group template based on all individual T_1 images in MNI space from both timepoints was created with Version 2.2.0 of the Advanced Normalization Tools (ANTs; Avants et al., 2017; Avants et al., 2011; Avants et al., 2010), following the method described in Cafiero et al. (2018).

7.2.5 *Surface based morphometry*

EXTRACTION OF CORTICAL SURFACE MEASURES.   Using the Computational Anatomy Toolbox (CAT12; Version r1109; Gaser & Dahnke, 2017) for SPM12 Update Revision Number 6906 (Friston et al., 2007; SPM12, 2016) in MATLAB Version

R2017b (The MathWorks, Inc., 2017), T_1 data in template space were segmented into grey and white matter.

For segmentation, study-specific paediatric tissue probability maps were generated using the Automated Segmentation Tool (Y. Zhang et al., 2001) as part of the FMRIB Software Library (FSL, Version 5.0; FMRIB Analysis Group, 2015). Tissue priors were derived from the common group template of both timepoints to account for the anatomical details of our developmental sample. Probability maps were normalised to sum to one. Finally, all maps were resampled to a resolution of 1.5mm isotropic and smoothed using a 35mm FWHM kernel, to approximate the resolution and smoothness of SPM's default anatomical priors. Additionally, grey and white matter maps created this way were used to replace the default template for the fast diffeomorphic image registration (DARTEL; Ashburner, 2007) procedure. For each participant, surface-based maps of cortical thickness (CT), gyrification index (GI; Lüders et al., 2006), cortical folding complexity (CF; Yotter, Nenadic, et al., 2011) and sulcus depth (SD) were extracted during segmentation. Following the matched-filter theorem, thickness data were smoothed with a 15mm FWHM kernel, and folding, gyrification and sulcus depth data were smoothed with a 20mm FWHM kernel.

QUANTIFYING DEVELOPMENTAL CORTICAL CHANGES.
The goal of the current study was to examine the relation between cortical surface plasticity and early numeracy abilities. To this end, participant-specific templates based on the

individual T_1 MNI images at both time points were generated using ANTs (Avants et al., 2017; Avants et al., 2011; Avants et al., 2010; Cafiero et al., 2018). Registration of a child's T_1 data to its respective template before segmentation and extraction of surface-based measures ensured optimal alignment for both time points. For each child, cortical change was quantified by subtracting the whole-brain maps of time point 1 from the whole-brain maps of time point 2, thus creating difference maps (Δ_{CT}, Δ_{GI}, Δ_{CF} and Δ_{SD}).

Additionally, we performed a ROI based analysis focused on areas previously linked to mathematical processing in adults and children: bilateral IPS, hippocampus (HIP), dorso-lateral prefrontal cortex (DLPFC), VTOC, and VWFA. ROIs are depicted in Figure 7.1.

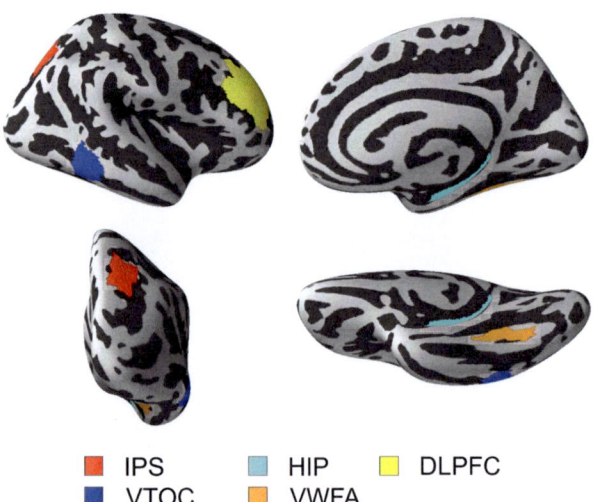

Figure 7.1: Overview of regions of interest. Only right-hemispheric regions are depicted, but bilateral regions were used in the analysis. IPS = intraparietal sulcus; VTOC = ventral temporal-occipital cortex; DLPFC = dorso-lateral prefrontal cortex; HIP = hippocampus; VWFA = visual word form area.

Participant-specific surface-based ROI masks were generated based on a multi-modal parcellation of brain areas comprising 180 cortical regions per hemisphere (Glasser et al., 2016). To this end, the parcellation was first spatially aligned with each child's MNI-T_1 volumetric image and then mapped to the respective participant's surface using the 'Map volume (Native Space) to individual surface' function in CAT12. The resulting ROIs in individual surface space served as masks to extract region-specific means of CT, GI, SD and CF for both time points. Finally, ROI-based cortical change from kindergarten to school was quantified by subtracting the mean of a region from time point 1 from the respective mean derived from time point 2 (school) for each participant, creating measures of Δ_{CT}, Δ_{GI}, Δ_{CF} and Δ_{SD}.

7.2.6 *Statistical analysis*

Whole-brain maps of Δ_{CT}, Δ_{GI}, Δ_{CF} and Δ_{SD} were correlated with the two subscales of the Heidelberg computation test (HRT; Haffner et al., 2005) using SPM12 (Update Revision Number 6906; Friston et al., 2007; SPM12, 2016). These subscales comprise a measure of (a) early arithmetic abilities and (b) visuospatial skills. Covariates included in the general linear models used for analysis were age at time 1, time between scans, sex, handedness, non-verbal IQ at time 2, maternal education, spelling accuracy, reading speed, and familial risk of developing dyslexia. To examine possible associations between brain maturation and the specific subscales, the respective other test score was added

Table 7.1: Overview of demographic information and psychometric performance of participants.

	Kindergarten	End of second grade
Demographic information		
N	28	28
Age[a]	5;6+6	8;5+5
Sex (male / female)	13/15	13/15
Maternal education[b]	4.43+0.51	..
Handedness[b]	58.11+44.63	..
Psychometric assessment	..	
Non-verbal IQ[c]	104.61+11.54	113.64+11.83
Arithmetic ability[d]	..	69.64+23.17
Numerical-logical / visu-ospatial abilities[d]	..	77.00+20.00
Spelling accuracy[d]	..	52.39+24.33
Reading speed[d]	..	63.71+24.96

[a] years; months, age at MRI-scan, mean + std in months
[b] measure only assessed at kindergarten age
[c] mean + standard deviation
[d] percentile ranks, mean + std; measure only assessed at school age

as a further covariate. We considered clusters to be significant when they exceeded a voxel-level threshold of $p < 0.001$ (un-corrected), with family-wise-error (FWE) correction for multiple spatial comparisons at the cluster level ($p < 0.05$).

Additionally, ROI-wise partial correlations of the z-transformed difference measures Δ_{CT}, Δ_{GI}, Δ_{CF} and Δ_{SD} with arithmetic abilities and visuospatial skills, respectively, were computed using R-3.3.1 (R Core Team, 2016). These correlations were corrected for the same confounding variables stated above. The ROI-based analysis was controlled for multiple comparisons

by correcting for number of ROIs (i. e. ten) and number of behavioural subscales (i. e. two). Consequently, ROI results are reported if $p < 0.0025$.

7.3   RESULTS

Information regarding participant's demographic data and performance in psychometric testing is provided in Table 7.1.

Our set of whole-brain analyses tested for clusters of significant correlation between cortical surface plasticity within CT, GI,
CF and SD and school-age visuospatial and arithmetic abilities.
Several clusters denoting associations between cortical change
and behavioural measures reached significance (see Table 7.2
and Figure 7.2). Specifically, CT plasticity was positively correlated with visuospatial skills in the right superior parietal lobe
(SPL; $R^2(16) = 0.74$, $p < 0.0001$) and the right precentral gyrus
($R^2(16) = 0.66$, $p = 0.0060$). Furthermore, CT change was negatively correlated with arithmetic abilities in the right temporal
pole (TP; $R^2(16) = 0.68$, $p = 0.0200$). Additionally, a negative correlation between CF change and visuospatial abilities reached
significance in a cluster within the right middle frontal gyrus
(MFG; $R^2(16) = 0.70$, $p = 0.0020$). Beyond the whole-brain results,
the ROI-based analysis revealed a significant negative correlation between change in CF and the arithmetic ability subscale
within the right IPS ($R^2(16) = 0.71$, $p = 0.0010$, Figure 7.3). No
further significant correlations were observed as part of the ROI
analysis.

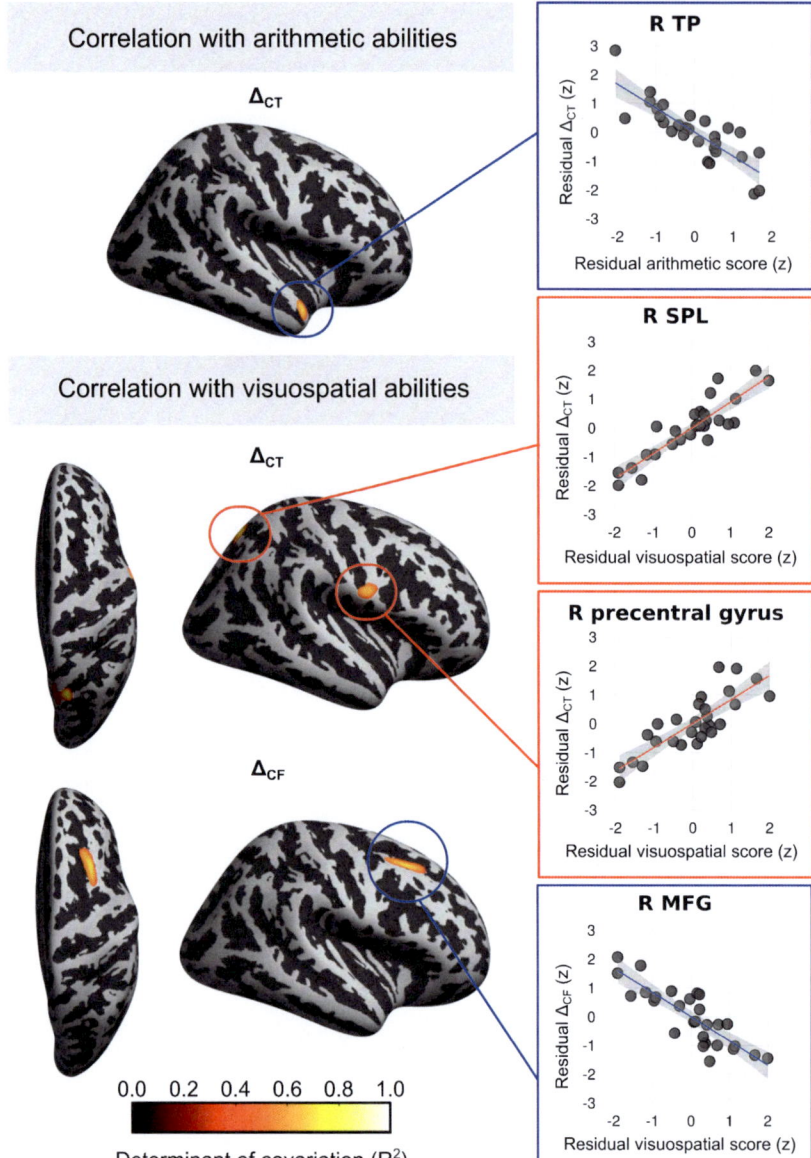

Figure 7.2: Overview of clusters denoting significant partial correlations of surface change and arithmetic (top row) and visuospatial abilities (middle and bottom). The color bar depicts the proportion of explained variance within each cluster in terms of the determinant of covariation (R^2), overlaid on the inflated cortical surfaces. (Continued on the following page.)

Figure 7.2 (cont.): Scatterplots show associations of the z-scored, maximal R^2 value of each residual cluster and the respective residual behavioral test score after removing the effects of age at kindergarten, time between scans, sex, handedness, non-verbal IQ at the end of second grade, maternal education, spelling accuracy, reading speed, familial risk of developing dyslexia, and the other subscale of the standardised math test (HRT). Shaded areas surrounding regression lines depict the respective 95% confidence level intervals. All reported results are significant at a level of $p < 0.05$ (family-wise-error corrected). Δ_{CT} = change in cortical thickness; Δ_{CF} = change in cortical folding complexity; R = right; TP = temporal pole; SPL = superior parietal lobe; MFG = middle frontal gyrus.

7.4   DISCUSSION

The second study of the present thesis examined associations between changes in cortical surface anatomy and emerging individual differences in arithmetic and visuospatial abilities—two essential components of numeracy—in typically developing children. Importantly, to identify anatomical correlates of numeracy skills specifically, particular care was taken to include pertinent covariates such as sociodemographic status and individual literacy performance. Unlike previous studies, the current analysis focused on developmental trajectories from kindergarten to school, when children start undergoing formal mathematical instruction. Developmental trajectories of different surface morphological measures were correlated with arithmetic and visuospatial magnitude processing performance derived from a standardised, age-normed math test conducted at the end of second grade in school.

The results revealed significant correlations of cortical surface plasticity with individual differences in primary school nu-

Table 7.2: Results of the whole brain surface-based morphometry analysis. The table provides and overview of clusters denoting significant partial correlations of surface change and arithmetic and visuospatial abilities, respectively.

	Coordinates			Size[a]	R^2	p^b
	x	y	z			
Arithmetic ability						
Δ_{CT}						
R temporal pole	50	14	-19	359	0.68	0.0200
Numerical-logical /						
visuo-spatial abilities						
Δ_{CF}						
R middle frontal gyrus	33	17	50	657	0.70	0.0020
Δ_{CF}						
R superior parietal cortex	18	-65	53	762	0.74	0.0001
R pre-/ postcentral gyrus	60	-2	17	462	0.66	0.0060

[a] size in vertices
[b] family-wise error corrected
Δ_{CT} = change in cortical thickness; Δ_{CF} = change in cortical folding complexity; R = right.

meracy ability in regions associated with early quantity processing, arithmetic problem solving and memory (**Hypothesis II.a**). Specifically, the analysis revealed significant positive associations between visuospatial magnitude processing and Δ_{CT} within the right SPL (**Hypothesis II.b**) and precentral gyrus. Additionally, we detected a significant negative correlation of visuospatial magnitude processing skills with Δ_{CF} within the right MFG. Further, there was a significant negative relationship between arithmetic performance and CT change in the right

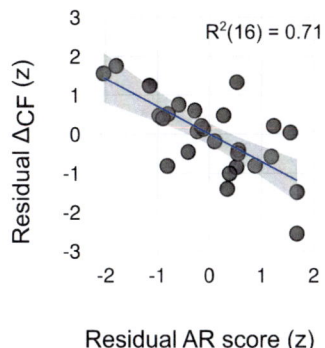

Figure 7.3: Partial correlation results of regions-of-interest analysis in the right IPS. The scatterplot illustrates the negative association between z-scored residual mean Δ_{CF} and residual arithmetic score in right IPS after removing the effects of age at kindergarten, time between scans, sex, handedness, non-verbal IQ at the end of second grade, maternal education, spelling accuracy, reading speed, familial risk of developing dyslexia, and the visuospatial magnitude processing score of the standardised math test (HRT). The shaded area surrounding the regression line depicts the 95% confidence level interval. Δ_{CF} = change in cortical folding complexity; AR = arithmetic.

temporal pole. Finally, the right IPS revealed a significant negative correlation between Δ_{CF} and symbolic arithmetic processing (**Hypothesis II.b**).

As discussed in Section 4.2, CT is a prominent measure for brain development and covaries systematically with the laminar structure of the cortex (Wagstyl & Lerch, 2018). However, as the relationship between the number of neurons and thickness of the cortex varies greatly across different brain areas (la Fougère et al., 2011), it is an unlikely marker of neuronal density. Rather, changes in this measure may be related to processes affecting the cytoarchitecture more generally. These may include glio- and synaptogenesis, synaptic pruning (Wagstyl & Lerch, 2018), and progressive white matter maturation of deep cortical layers (Natu et al., 2018). CF during development has been suggested to be driven by compression forces induced by sustained growth of the outer cortical surface, as neurons mature and form connections (Budday et al., 2015a, 2015b; Richman, Stewart, Hutchinson, & Caviness, 1975). Therefore, a possible explanation may be that observed differences reflect differential myelination and synaptic remodelling (Blanton et al., 2001).

Semantic and episodic memory associated with the medial and anterior temporal lobe are important neurocognitive processes supporting numeracy, e.g. in terms of storage and retrieval of number facts and knowledge of mathematical concepts (Menon, 2010). The vital role of the temporal lobe regions for sound numeracy development was further highlighted by reports of variable cortical structure within this area in dyscalculic children and adolescents (Ranpura et al., 2013). In line with this notion, our results suggest that neuroplastic change in the right temporal pole fulfils a seminal role for early mathematical development. Specifically, its change in CT was negatively associated with arithmetic performance. As a multimodal assocation area, the right anterior temporal pole supports integration of conceptual information from distributed regions (Patterson, Nestor, & Rogers, 2007). During neurotypical development, the anterior temporal lobe has been associated with a steady decline of CT (Ducharme et al., 2016; Fjell et al., 2015). Therefore, the positive link between reduced change and better arithmetic abilities observed in the current study might indicate a decreased rate of cortical thinning in well-performing children. Consequently, this might reflect sustained synaptogenesis within the semantic and episodic memory system during more successful mathematical learning.

Second, the posterior SPL has been associated with visuospatial processing across domains. For instance, Simon et al. (2002) report common superior parietal activation for tasks involving grasping, pointing, saccadic and visual attention orienting. Additionally, this region is assumed to house representations of the remembered orientation of visual stimuli (Ester et al., 2015). At the same time, the SPL is involved in adult numerical cognition in terms of counting (Knops et al., 2009; Piazza et al., 2002) and mathematical operations (Rosenberg-Lee et al., 2011). Remarkably, the right SPL supports approximate calculation already in preschool children (Cantlon et al., 2006).

In line with **Hypothesis II.b**, the current findings complement these data by suggesting a fundamental contribution of SPL plasticity for the refining visuospatial magnitude skills from kindergarten to school. In parietal regions such as the SPL, CT typically increases between five and eight years of age, before subsequently declining later in life (Ducharme et al., 2016; Shaw et al., 2008). The positive association of thickness change and mathematical ability might therefore suggest that increased synaptogenesis supports development of visuospatial skills in the first school years.

Not anticipated by the hypotheses of the current study, there was an additional positive association between visuospatial processing skills and CT change of the right lateral precentral gyrus,

an area typically associated with cortical thinning over development (Ducharme et al., 2016). Precentral regions have been previously linked to working memory processes that might play
a supportive role on mathematical cognition by refreshing visuospatial short-term representations (Menon, 2015). Following
this speculative interpretation, it is important to note that right
precentral regions are involved in tasks requiring spatial working memory rehearsal processes (E. E. Smith & Jonides, 1998). In
line with this finding, the present result might suggest a link between visuospatial processing skills and more rapid growth of
intracortical white matter indicated by increased rates of cortical
thinning within the precentral gyrus.

Further, better visuospatial performance was associated with
reduced change in the regularity of cortical folding within the
prefrontal cortex, specifically the right MFG (**Hypothesis I.a**).
Previous studies emphasises the role of this region for working memory, thus supporting numerical cognition. For instance,
Menon, Rivera, White, Glover, and Reiss (2000) report involvement of the MFG during calculation tasks with increased working memory demands in adult participants. In line with this,
Rotzer et al. (2008) link the working-memory deficits specific
to numerical processing in children with dyscalculia to reduced
grey-matter volume in bilateral MFG. The rate of plasticity of
gyral convolutions might be driven by differential synaptogenesis within outer cortical layers across individuals (Budday et al.,
2015a, 2015b). Therefore, children with better visuospatial mag-

nitude processing skills might exhibit more mature intracortical synaptic connectivity in the right MFG early on.

Finally, the ROI analysis revealed a negative association between folding plasticity if the right IPS and arithmetic ability (**Hypotheses II.a, II.b**), indicating less folding change for well-performing children. The right IPS is known as a key region for the development of typical numerical cognition. In children as young as four years of age, magnitude processing is related to right-lateralised parietal activation (Cantlon et al., 2006). With development of symbolic arithmetic processing skills during later childhood and adolescence, involvement of left parietal regions increases (Rivera et al., 2005). The degree of this functional shift, however, seems to be related to the individual level of competence: Individuals that perform poorly in maths persistently recruit the right IPS, even during simple arithmetic tasks (De Smedt, Holloway, & Ansari, 2011; G. R. Price, Mazzocco, & Ansari, 2013). In view of these findings, the current results indicate that successful mathematical learning is related to more mature intracortical synaptic connectivity of the right IPS at an early age. Thus, more stable magnitude representations might support acquisition of efficient basic processing strategies.

Contrary to the expectation formulated in **Hypothesis II.a**, the current analysis did not identify any numeracy-related structural plasticity within the MTL. This was somewhat surprising, given the prominently reported role of MTL regions during mathematical development. For instance, Qin et al. (2014) demonstrated an age-related increase in hippocampal involvement in children from seven to nine years of age, associated with an increased use of memory-based fact retrieval strategies for solving simple arithmetic tasks. Furthermore, Supekar et al. (2013) showed that initial hippocampal volume predicts behavioural improvement in mathematics following an intense eight-week math tutoring program. In stark contrast to these accounts, the present results suggest a less important role of the MTL memory system at a younger age when children first undergo formal mathematical instruction. Instead, the results of the current study emphasise the role of areas involved in working memory, visuospatial processing and basic representation of magnitude. Nevertheless, it is impossible to rule out any functional contributions of the MTL during this time from the structural analysis presented here. Future investigations are necessary to examine the functional organisation of emerging mathematical abilities from kindergarten to school age.

Taken together, Empirical Study II links cortical surface plasticity to numeracy learning during the first years of formal mathematical instruction in school. The results reveal associations between specific trajectories of structural reorganisation and emerging arithmetic and visuospatial magnitude skills, respectively. Thereby, this study highlights the role of regions associated with working memory, basic magnitude processing, semantic memory and visuospatial processing, identifying early cortical surface plasticity as the structural brain basis of emerging numeracy abilities during the first years of school.

CHAPTER 8

GENERAL DISCUSSION

This final chapter will focus on summarising the results of the two empirical studies presented in this thesis (Section 8.1) and provide a general discussion on how they corroborate and expand the current understanding of literacy deficits and numeracy acquisition.

Specifically, Section 8.2 will put the results of the experiment described in Chapter 6 in context with prominent neurobiological theories of DD. Subsequently, Section 8.3 incorporates the findings of the second empirical study presented in Chapter 7 with previous neuroimaging research in the field of numeracy and mathematical cognition. Finally, the present thesis closes with some concluding remarks in Section 8.4.

8.1 SUMMARY OF RESULTS

The current thesis was designed with the aim to examine specific neural correlates of deficient literacy acquisition and individual differences in numeracy attainment. Consequently, the two studies presented here targeted research questions concerning (a) neural differences distinguishing future dyslexic children from typically developing controls before and after literacy in-struction in school and (b) specific developmental trajectories of brain surface anatomy between five and eight years of age as-sociated with individual numeracy attainment. Both questions were investigated using longitudinal data acquired from chil-dren undergoing a comprehensive series of psychometric testing and neuroimaging from kindergarten until the end of second grade in school. Following participants over this period of time revealed specific neurobiological profiles related to individual behavioural variation. Specifically, the presented analysis quan-tified diverse neuroanatomical and -functional measures, while controlling for pertinent covariates including sociodemographic status, intellectual abilities and individual performance in liter-acy and numeracy.

The focus of **Empirical Study I** presented in Chapter 6 was a systematic investigation of neural origins of DD, a prominent neurodevelopmental disorder. There is much debate concerning the underlying causal neurological deficits due to its heteroge-nous nature (see Section 2.1.2.1). Importantly, comprehensive data of preliterate dyslexic children is sparse and previous stud-ies often paid little attention to comprehensively control for co-morbidities and confounding factors such as mathematical abil-ity or socio-economic status. Consequently, while also taking these factors into account, I systematically examined the involve-ment of complex cortical and subcortical networks assumed to play a causal role for the emergence of literacy deficits by com-bining resting-state fMRI, T_1- and diffusion-weighted imaging.

The results show converging evidence for cortical malformation and reduced functional coherence within the speech processing system. Specifically, future dyslexics' left primary auditory cortex was characterised by higher degrees of CF both before and after first formal literacy instruction. Additionally, transient differences between children that developed DD later in life and those who acquired literacy effortlessly were detected when comparing structural and functional connectivity of left perisylvian regions. These effects include increased connectivity strength of the arcuate fasciculus connecting the planum temporale and BA6 and reduced functional connectivity between the left primary auditory cortex and the planum temporale. In conclusion, these findings contribute to our understanding of the nature of a phonological deficit ultimately hampering literacy learning in dyslexia.

So far, little was known regarding neural correlates of individual achievement in early numeracy abilities acquired within the first two years of school. Therefore, **Empirical Study II** was designed to investigate trajectories of cortical development specifically related to these skills, while accounting for individual levels of literacy achievement. Specifically, correlations between cortical surface plasticity from the last year of kindergarten until the second grade in school and performance in arithmetic and visuospatial magnitude processing tasks at eight years of age were analysed. The results reveal a link between these two fundamental aspects of basic numeracy and cortical surface reorganisation within right-hemispheric regions. Specifically, arithmetic abilities significantly correlated with CF plasticity of the right intraparietal sulcus and CT of the anterior temporal pole. At the same time, visuospatial magnitude processing skills were significantly associated with changes in CT within the right superior parietal lobe and the precentral gyrus, as well as with CF plasticity of the middle frontal gyrus. Overall, these results reveal a connection of emerging numeracy skills and structural reorganisation of regions known to support visuospatial processing, working memory and semantic memory.

8.2   INTEGRATING THE CURRENT FINDINGS WITH THEORIES OF DEVELOPMENTAL DYSLEXIA

Section 2.1.2.1 highlights the disagreement within the literature regarding the aetiology of DD. This disagreement is sparked by the broad range of behavioural variability in terms of atypical phonological, low-level sensory, and motor processing exhibited by dyslexic individuals. Additionally, the equally inconsistent neurobiological evidence provided by numerous studies over decades of research supplies further fuel for this debate. Developmental evidence, tracing atypical behavioural and neural profiles of dyslexic individuals from early in life, offers the potential to disentangle possible causes from consequences of DD to get to the root of the deficit.

The multimodal MRI assessment presented in Chapter 6 clearly points towards a phonological deficit at the core of literacy problems in the children participating in our study. Importantly, the results presented here extend the currently sparse evidence of neuroanatomical anomalies within the speech processing system of preliterate dyslexic children (Clark et al., 2014), by providing a thorough analysis of cortical surface morphometry, white matter connectivity and resting-state functional coherence. Thereby, the data supports the prominent phonological deficit theory (Vellutino et al., 2004). According to this account, poor phonological skills hinder beginning readers to form associations between letters and their corresponding sounds, impeding fluent literacy attainment (Snowling, 1998).

Importantly, the current neuroimaging results are in line with the behavioural profile exhibited by future dyslexic children in our study, emphasising the role of deficient speech sound processing. This behavioural variation is well-established in the literature, with phonological awareness—followed by phonological short-term memory and rapid automatised naming—most reliably distinguishing cases from controls already before literacy instruction (Moll, Kunze, et al., 2014; Ziegler et al., 2010). These observations are in line with a considerable body of previous neuroanatomical research in older participants past the age of initial literacy acquisition, from early post-mortem histological work (Galaburda et al., 1985), over evidence from structural neuroimaging (Richlan et al., 2013), to studies reporting aberrant white matter structure within the dorsal reading network (Saygin et al., 2013; Vandermosten et al., 2012). Additionally, they complement foregone functional work suggesting abnormal spectro-temporal analysis of speech (Lehongre et al., 2011) contingent on the same areas exhibiting faulty cross-talk in the present study (Giraud & Poeppel, 2012).

Observed differences between future dyslexic children and controls at a preliterate age encompass different aspects such as gyrification, functional connectivity and streamline density within the dorsal reading network. Based on the data at hand, however, it is impossible to say whether these effects arise concomitantly over development. In fact, it may be that one acts as a primary deficit causing the other differences already at a pre-reading age. A likely—though speculative—scenario could be that atypical gyrification of the primary auditory cortex and disrupted functional coherence between regions within Heschl's gyrus mark aberrant neural migration. Especially gyrification is a measure that typically undergoes only very little change after the first years of life (Li et al., 2014; T. White et al., 2010), strongly pointing to malformations during pre- or perinatal neuronal development (Bayly et al., 2014; Mutlu et al., 2013). Consequently, the observed differences in streamline density might present a secondary result arising from compensatory articulatory recoding strategies supported by the ventral premotor cortex (see Figure 8.1; Pugh et al., 2000; Richlan et al., 2011; S. E. Shaywitz et al., 1998).

To draw a comprehensive picture of neural precursors of DD, fibre pathways and areas beyond the phonological domain were examined. However, no significant differences between cases and controls were detected in subcortical sensory processing regions, ventral occipitotemporal cortex or the cerebellum. Thus,

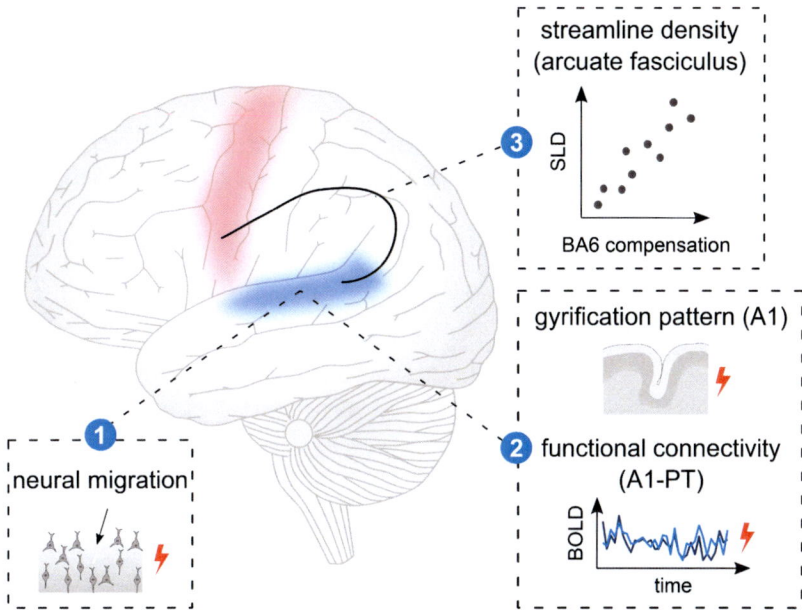

Figure 8.1: Putative developmental scenario underlying differences
observed in preliterate children that developed dyslexia.
Neural migration defects reported in post-mortem data
within left perisylvian regions (Panel 1; Galaburda & Kemper, 1979; Galaburda et al., 1985) might lead to the present
findings of aberrant gyrification within the left primary
auditory cortex and disrupted functional connectivity between the primary auditory cortex and the planum temporale (Panel 2). As a consequence, dyslexic individuals may
rely more on articulatory recoding strategies supported
by the ventral premotor cortex (BA 6; Pugh et al., 2000;
Richlan et al., 2011; S. E. Shaywitz et al., 1998). This increased compensatory activity might in turn strengthen the
structure of the interconnecting arcuate fasciculus, leading
to the observed increase in streamline density (Panel 3). A1
= primary auditory cortex; PT = planum temporale; SLD =
sreamline density; BA6 = Brodmann area 6; red region =
BA6; blue region = superior temporal gyrus.

our data fails to provide support for corresponding theories

claiming respective deficits to be at the root of DD (see Table 6.1).

While the results presented in this thesis support the phono-

logical deficit theory of DD, the lack of evidence for non-

phonological impairments has to be taken with the care generally devoted to null effects. This could imply one of several alternative scenarios that cannot be disentangled here. For instance, it might be that deficits supposed in most prominent neural accounts beyond the phonological theory are indeed consequences of impoverished literacy experience and thus a side effect of living a life with DD (Huettig et al., 2018).

A second feasible interpretation regards the possibility that there are several independent neural profiles leading to literacy deficits. This notion aligns with the account of distinct cognitive subgroups of dyslexia provided by Stefan Heim et al. (2008) (see also Pennington et al., 2012). In fact, Jednoróg, Gawron, Marchewka, Heim, and Grabowska (2014) reported distinct variations in cortical volume for groups with different behavioural phenotypes in 10-year-old dyslexic children and adults. In the light of this subgroup-account, it would be highly remarkable that our sample predominantly included children with the phonological subtype while no such focus was placed during the recruiting procedure. Nevertheless, this scenario could account for dyslexic cases that do not exhibit phonological processing deficits (Bosse et al., 2007; Peyrin et al., 2012), an otherwise substantial limitation of the results presented here.

A third possibility concerns the fact that the power of our study was too limited to pick up more subtle differences, even though the number of dyslexic cases included in the analysis was comparable if not superior to previous work. However, it cannot be ruled out that—given a larger, behaviourally more heterogenous sample—further differences might emerge.

To disentangle these possibilities, subsequent studies are required adapting the experimental design employed here at an even grander scale. Work based on a larger population of dyslexic children will offer higher levels of statistical power. An even more comprehensive assessment of behavioural characteristics (e. g. also measuring individual motoric abilities) would further add to our understanding of possible behavioural phenotypes present in DD. Additionally, future studies are needed to evaluate the generalisability of the current results to other, non-alphabetic or less transparent writing systems. Further, following children over an even more extended amount of time would permit to characterise the progression of atypical brain development that also arises as a consequence of literacy deficits.

In conclusion, **Empricial study I** adds to the understanding of neural precursors of DD. While the presented results cannot give unequivocal proof that impairments in speech sound processing are the sole underlying cause, they highlight phonological deficits as a significant contributor to the dyslexic phenotype. What is more, they describe a disruption of the phonological system in terms of early auditory cortex malformation and aberrant downstream connectivity, thus indicating a fundamental neural deficit that hampers successful literacy learning.

8.3   INTEGRATING CURRENT FINDINGS WITH THEORIES OF NUMERACY DEVELOPMENT

Empirical Study II addresses an important research gap in the literature by shedding light onto the associations between cortical surface plasticity from kindergarten to school and early numeracy skills. Controlling for pertinent covariates such as literacy abilities and sociodemographic status, the results of the presented analysis reveal specific correlates of individual numeracy attainment, thus complementing the existing neurobiological accounts.

Importantly, insights about the structural and functional reorganisation supporting numeracy maturation are often derived from school age children that already master the first basic mathematical concepts. As explained in Section 2.2, a common picture emerges from these data: In addition to recruitment of core magnitude processing areas in the right PPC, immature processing seems to be related to greater reliance on regions associated with auxiliary functions including working memory and attention (i. e. PFC regions; Rivera et al., 2005). With age and experience, the contribution of these processes to numerical cognition diminishes, while the functional specialisation of the left PPC increases (Rivera et al., 2005). In line with this notion, left parietal grey matter volume at eight years of age, alongside prefrontal and ventral temporal regions, reliably predicts the longitudinal gain in mathematical abilities until adolescence (Evans et al., 2015). Additionally, involvement of MTL during mathematical processing initially increases, followed by a decrease in the course of adolescence (Qin et al., 2014). This trajectory has been associated with the initial development and subsequent consolidation of memory-based retrieval strategies that are more efficient than procedural approaches for mathematical problem solving (Ashcraft, 1982; Barrouillet & Fayol, 1998; Qin et al., 2014; Siegler & Shipley, 1995). Consistent with this view, variable neural representations in MTL distinguish children that rely more on retrieval from those who employ procedural strategies (Cho et al., 2011).

The results of **Empirical Study II** presented in this thesis shed light onto structural reorganisation processes occurring at an even earlier stage before the above-mentioned changes occur (see Figure 8.2). In doing so, the current results reveal differential contributions of right PPC regions to distinct subcomponents of numeracy skill, namely arithmetic and visuospatial magnitude processing abilities. Specifically, cortical surface reorganisation in terms of cortical folding within the IPS was related to individual performance in arithmetic. Plasticity of cortical thickness within the SPL was related to behavioural differences in visuospatial magnitude processing. This distinction lends new support from a very young age group to the tripartite model of parietal contributions for numerical processing formulated by Dehaene et al. (2003). In this model, the IPS is characterised as a domain specific region housing the core magnitude representations equivalent to concept of the mental number line, crucial for stable neural representations and thus successful mathematical

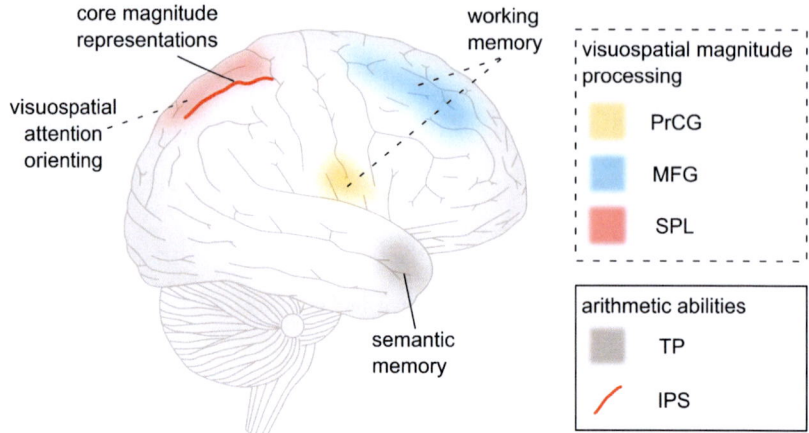

Figure 8.2: Regions of longitudinal neuroplastic change relevant for emerging numeracy skills, as identified in **Empirical Study II** of this thesis. Labels on the brain denote functions individual regions were associated with in previous literature (for core magnitude representations and visuospatual attention orienting, see Dehaene et al., 2003; for working memory, see Menon et al., 2000; E. E. Smith and Jonides, 1998; for semantic memory, see Menon et al., 2000; Patterson et al., 2007). Boxes on the right denote which region's neuroplastic change from kindergarten to primary school was related to either visuospatial magnitude processing (top) or arithmetic abilities (bottom). PrCG = precentral gyrus; MFG = middle frontal gyrus; SPL = superior parietal lobe; TP = temporal pole; IPS = intraparietal sulcus.

learning. In contrast, the SPL is characterised as an area involved in visuospatial attention orienting, thereby supporting visuospatial magnitude processing (see Figure 8.2).

Based on the reported associations between specific parietal surface trajectories and differential mathematical and visuospatial performance, it could conceivably be hypothesised that parietal plasticity differentiates groups of well-performing from poorly performing children already at an early age. Further support for such a hypothesis comes from accounts of deficient parietal processing in older children and adults with developmental

dyscalculia (Mussolin et al., 2009; G. R. Price, Holloway, Räsänen, Vesterinen, & Ansari, 2007). Taken together with the current
results, these deficits might potentially be rooted in structural
parietal malformations. This hypothesis might be addressed in
future studies with larger sample sizes, also including individuals with severe deficits in mathematical learning.

Beyond parietal contributions to emerging numeracy abilities,
the current results highlight the role of regions associated with
more domain-general, auxiliary processes during early numeracy attainment. Observed effects were located in regions associated with working memory processing, i. e. the right MFG
(Menon et al., 2000) and the right precentral gyrus (E. E. Smith
& Jonides, 1998). There is a large number of studies demonstrating that working memory explains a substantial proportion of
the variance of individual performance in mathematical tasks,
both in typically developing children and those that experience
difficulties in numeracy processing (Raghubar, Barnes, & Hecht,
2010). Thus, the current results provide insights into structural
correlates of this working memory contribution at the transition
from kindergarten to school age, when children first undergo
formal mathematical instruction.

While previous work in older children consistently ascer-
tained contributions of the MTL to the development of numerical cognition (Cho et al., 2011; Qin et al., 2014; Rivera et al., 2005),
no association between emerging numeracy abilities and medial temporal surface plasticity was identified for our younger
study sample. This may put a new perspective on the current

understanding of developmental trajectories involved in the maturation of early numerical cognition. Typically, MTL correlates are interpreted to reflect the development of memory-based retrieval strategies based on the consolidation of mathematical knowledge (Ashcraft, 1982; Barrouillet & Fayol, 1998; Qin et al., 2014; Siegler & Shipley, 1995). The current data, however, suggest that initial formal mathematical learning is predominantly supported by plasticity in core magnitude and working memory regions and does not provide evidence for a putative role of memory processes within the MTL. Importantly, as a null finding, this lack of evidence does not permit to draw conclusions about the involvement of memory-based processing at such an early stage in mathematical development. Rather, it opens up an avenue for future research to examine if structural reorganisation of the MTL gradually emerges as a function of individual problem-solving strategies. Children in second grade—the age when our sample was tested—are reported to predominantly rely on procedural counting strategies (Barrouillet & Fayol, 1998; Qin et al., 2014; Siegler & Shipley, 1995). Via thorough assessment of distinct approaches used by individual children, future studies may shed light onto the association between plasticity of the MTL and emerging mathematical competence, also across a more extended age range as presented here.

Overall, it is noteworthy that all significant effects reported in **Empirical Study II** were confined to the right hemisphere. This is in stark contrast to the results presented by Evans et al. (2015), who showed that gain in arithmetic abilities could be predicted from intrinsic connectivity and grey matter volume within left-sided areas of the arithmetic network at eight years of age. This lends support to the hypothesis that right-hemispheric processes promote initial numeracy development, while involvement of left hemispheric regions increases with age and experience (Rivera et al., 2005).

Despite providing information about intrinsic associations between cortical surface plasticity and individual behavioural performance, it is important to stress that the results presented here are purely correlational, such that causation cannot be inferred. Consequently, from these results we cannot disentangle whether behavioural changes drive neuroanatomical variation or vice versa.

In conclusion, **Empirical Study II** provides evidence highlighting the little-known associations between cortical surface reorganisation from kindergarten to school age and individual numeracy skills. The insights obtained from this study complement previous work investigating the relationship between brain maturation and numerical cognition in older children. Specifically, the results provide support for the importance of specific developmental trajectories in confined, right-hemispheric areas promoting core magnitude, visuospatial and memory processing at the transition from kindergarten to school, when children first undergo formal mathematical instruction.

8.4   CONCLUDING REMARKS

In the scope of this thesis, I examined the brain basis of complex cognitive abilities—i. e. literacy and numeracy—using structural and resting-state functional MRI data longitudinally obtained from young children. Combining longitudinal neuroimaging and extensive psychometric testing in children from kindergarten to school, the results shed light onto neural correlates of (*a*) deficient literacy acquisition in DD and (*b*) individual differences in mathematical development.

Thereby, the work reported in the current thesis overcomes prominent shortcomings in the literature: Based on a longitudinal design, neural correlates identified before the start of school are less likely to be confounded by individual variations in literacy and numeracy experience. Assessing both literacy and numeracy abilities, the considerable covariation between these domains was accounted for. Combining measures of cortical surface geometry, white matter structure and resting-state functional coherence, a more complete characterisation of the variable neuroanatomical and -functional profiles through development could be achieved.

By controlling for prominent covariates including measures of the respective other domain, specific associations between neural development and literacy and numeracy were revealed. Consequently, this thesis does not engage with identifying the common neural basis of these complex cognitive functions and their deficits. Even though beyond the scope of the current work, such an undertaking would be certainly worthwhile. To obtain a complete developmental picture of these processes and their deficits, children that will go on to develop either isolated dyslexia, dyscalculia, or co-occurring deficits in both domains together with typical controls would need to be assessed as early as possible. Adapting a longitudinal design, children should be continuously assessed starting from pre-school and continuing throughout the first years of their academic career. Despite the relatively high prevalence rates of dyslexia and dyscalculia, this is hard to achieve: it is unclear how many children recruited before schooling will develop deficits, so it is impossible to determine how many cases will be included in the final set. Furthermore, developmental neuroimaging work is often riddled with high drop-out rates due to lack of compliance or disrupted data quality especially for young children. One of the rare studies looking at such a unique sample of children aged seven to 12 years was reported by (Skeide et al., 2018), who describe a distinct neuroanatomical and -functional profile centred on the right parahippocampal gyrus for children with co-occurring difficulties, providing a first theoretical framework as a possible basis for future work.

Still, the current sample grants valuable insights into the emergence of literacy deficits and numeracy skills. Together, the results of both studies present a strong case for more comprehensive analyses of cortical surface anatomy as a valuable addition to classical measures such as GMV and CT. Importantly, both gyrification and CF were identified as region-specific early correlates of literacy outcome and individual numeracy skills. This may be taken as an important implication for developmental psychology, as cellular mechanisms that underly the emergence of complex cognitive behaviour may profoundly shape the brain's anatomy across various dimensions. Thus, while future investigations are necessary to validate the microanatomical underpinnings of differential cortical surface development, these measures may provide more detailed insights into the brain's anatomy and its intricate relationship with cognition (Mechelli et al., 2005; Rivera et al., 2005).

As emphasised in Section 2.3, the empirical work presented in the current thesis comprises two studies investigating specific neural correlates of early literacy deficits and emerging numeracy skills. Importantly, in all analyses behavioural variation in the respective other domain was taken into account. Integrating the current results of both studies highlights the importance of distinct core processes for sound literacy and numeracy learning, respectively. The findings of **Empirical Study I** revealed the severe ramifications of disruptions within confined cortical circuits supporting phonological processing within the dorsal reading network for literacy acquisition. The data presented in **Empirical Study II**, in contrast, underlines the role of plasticity within parietal regions specifically involved in magnitude processing for early mathematical performance. What is more, previous literature suggested parietal dysfunction in older children and adults with developmental dyscalculia (Mussolin et al., 2009; G. R. Price et al., 2007; Rotzer et al., 2008), even though it remains to be shown whether this also holds for young children who struggle with numeracy at the transition from kindergarten to school. Nevertheless, a common picture that seems to hold for both literacy and numeracy skills is the reliance on separate core processes supported by distinct neural circuitries. Consequently, specific disturbances of these core faculties may be the most likely candidates for a neural basis of isolated deficits in the respective domains.

However, it is important to note that these core processes do not seem to operate in isolation. Evidence for the importance of auxiliary functions—most notably working memory—needed to acquire complex cognitive abilities like numeracy is provided by the results of **Empirical Study II**. While an empirical assessment of domain-general faculties supporting successful literacy acquisition was beyond the scope of the current work, it could be conceivably hypothesised that processes like working memory, in concert with executive functioning (Yeniad et al., 2013), focused attention (Lundberg & Sterner, 2006) and visual associative learning (Skeide et al., 2018) constitute a common cognitive basis for both emerging literacy and numeracy skills in typically developing children.

In the introduction of this thesis, I set out with the question for the specific neural origins of differences in emerging complex cognitive abilities. Consequently, the current work— shedding light onto the developmental trajectories underlying literacy deficits and numeracy development—makes a substantial step towards a more comprehensive understanding how complex cognitive skills emerge and how specific disruptions may cause learning deficits. The presented evidence suggests that acquisition and maturation of these abilities reshapes the circuitries for domain-specific as well as domain-general auxiliary functions (i.e. magnitude, visuospatial and working memory processing in numeracy), and that disruptions in regions supporting very specific aspects of complex processes have severe consequences for learning (i.e. disruptions of the phonological systems impeding literacy development).

BIBLIOGRAPHY

Alm, J., & Andersson, J. (1997). A study of literacy in prisons in Uppsala. *Dyslexia*, *3*(4), 245–246.

Amalric, M., & Dehaene, S. (2016). Origins of the brain networks for advanced mathematics in expert mathematicians. *Proceedings of the National Academy of Sciences of the United States of America*, *113*(18), 4909–4917.

Amitay, S., Ben-Yehudah, G., Banai, K., & Ahissar, M. (2002). Disabled readers suffer from visual and auditory impairments but not from a specific magnocellular deficit. *Brain*, *125*(10), 2272–2285.

Amlien, I. K., Fjell, A. M., Tamnes, C. K., Grydeland, H., Krogsrud, S. K., Chaplin, T. A., . . . Walhovd, K. B. (2016). Organizing principles of human cortical development—Thickness and area from 4 to 30 Years: Insights from comparative primate neuroanatomy. *Cerebral Cortex*, *26*(1), 257–267.

Andersson, J. L. R., Skare, S., & Ashburner, J. T. (2003). How to correct susceptibility distortions in spin-echo echo-planar images: Application to diffusion tensor imaging. *NeuroImage*, *20*(2), 870–888.

Ansari, D., & Dhital, B. (2006). Age-related changes in the activation of the intraparietal sulcus during nonsymbolic magnitude processing: An event-related functional magnetic resonance imaging study. *Journal of Cognitive Neuroscience*, *18*(11), 1820–1828.

Ansari, D., Dhital, B., & Siong, S. C. (2006). Parametric effects of numerical distance on the intraparietal sulcus during passive viewing of rapid numerosity changes. *Brain Research*, *1067*(1), 181–188.

Armstrong, E., Schleicher, A., Omran, H., Curtis, M., & Zilles, K. (1995). The ontogeny of human gyrification. *Cerebral Cortex*, *5*(1), 56–63.

Ashburner, J. T. (2007). A fast diffeomorphic image registration algorithm. *NeuroImage*, *38*(1), 95–113.

Ashburner, J. T., & Friston, K. J. (1997). Multimodal image coregistration and partitioning – A unified framework. *NeuroImage*, *6*(3), 209–217.

Ashburner, J. T., & Friston, K. J. (2000). Voxel-Based Morphometry – The methods. *NeuroImage*, *11*(6), 805–821.

Ashburner, J. T., & Friston, K. J. (2005). Unified segmentation. *NeuroImage*, *26*(3), 839–851.

Ashcraft, M. H. (1982). The development of mental arithmetic: A chronometric approach. *Developmental Review*, *2*(3), 213–236.

Avants, B. B., Tustison, N. J., & Johnson, H. J. (2017). Advanced Normalization Tools. Retrieved from http://stnava.github.io/ANTs/

Avants, B. B., Tustison, N. J., Song, G., Cook, P. A., Klein, A., & Gee, J. C. (2011). A reproducible evaluation of ANTs similarity metric performance in brain image registration. *NeuroImage, 54*(3), 2033–2044.

Avants, B. B., Yushkevich, P., Pluta, J., Minkoff, D., Korczykowski, M., Detre, J., & Gee, J. C. (2010). The optimal template effect in hippocampus studies of diseased populations. *NeuroImage, 49*(3), 2457–2466.

Azevedo, F. A. C., Carvalho, L. R. B., Grinberg, L. T., Farfel, J. M., Ferretti, R. E. L., Leite, R. E. P., ... Herculano-Houzel, S. (2009). Equal numbers of neuronal and nonneuronal cells make the human brain an isometrically scaled-up primate brain. *Journal of Comparative Neurology, 513*(5), 532–541.

Badian, N. A. (1999). Persistent arithmetic, reading, or arithmetic and reading disability. *Annals of Dyslexia, 49*(1), 43–70.

Baldeweg, T., Richardson, A., Watkins, S., Foale, C., & Gruzelier, J. (1999). Impaired auditory frequency discrimination in dyslexia detected with mismatch evoked potentials. *Annals of Neurology, 45*(4), 495–503.

Barateiro, A., & Fernandes, A. (2014). Temporal oligodendrocyte lineage progression: In vitro models of proliferation, differentiation and myelination. *Biochimica et Biophysica Acta (BBA) - Molecular Cell Research, 1843*(9), 1917–1929.

Barbiero, C., Lonciari, I., Montico, M., Monasta, L., Penge, R., Vio, C., ... Ronfani, L. (2012). The submerged dyslexia iceberg: How many school children are not diagnosed? Results from an Italian study. *PLOS ONE, 7*(10), e48082.

Barnea-Goraly, N., Menon, V., Eckert, M., Tamm, L., Bammer, R., Karchemskiy, A., ... Reiss, A. L. (2005). White matter development during childhood and adolescence: A cross-sectional diffusion tensor imaging study. *Cerebral Cortex, 15*(12), 1848–1854.

Barrouillet, P., & Fayol, M. (1998). From algorithmic computing to direct retrieval: Evidence from number and alphabetic arithmetic in children and adults. *Memory & Cognition, 26*(2), 355–368.

Barth, H., La Mont, K., Lipton, J. S., Dehaene, S., Kanwisher, N., & Spelke, E. S. (2006). Non-symbolic arithmetic in adults and young children. *Cognition, 98*, 199–222.

Barth, H., La Mont, K., Lipton, J., & Spelke, E. S. (2005). Abstract number and arithmetic in preschool children. *Proceedings of the National Academy of Sciences of the United States of America, 102*(39), 14116–14121.

Bartley, A. J., Jones, D. W., & Weinberger, D. R. (1997). Genetic variability of human brain size and cortical gyral patterns. *Brain, 120*(2), 257–269.

Bayly, P. V., Okamoto, R. J., Xu, G., Shi, Y., & Taber, L. A. (2013). A cortical folding model incorporating stress-dependent growth explains gyral wavelengths and stress patterns in the developing brain. *Physical Biology, 10*(1), 016005.

Bayly, P. V., Taber, L. A., & Kroenke, C. D. (2014). Mechanical forces in cerebral cortical folding: A review of measurements and models. *Journal of the Mechanical Behavior of Biomedical Materials, 29*, 568–581.

Behrens, T. E. J., Johansen-Berg, H., Jbabdi, S., Rushworth, M. F. S., & Woolrich, M. W. (2007). Probabilistic diffusion tractography with multiple fibre orientations: What can we gain? *NeuroImage, 34*(1), 144–155.

Behrens, T. E. J., Woolrich, M. W., Jenkinson, M., Johansen-Berg, H., Nunes, R. G., Clare, S., ... Smith, S. M. (2003). Characterization and propagation of uncertainty in diffusion-weighted MR imaging. *Magnetic Resonance in Medicine, 50*(5), 1077–1088.

Behzadi, Y., Restom, K., Liau, J., & Liu, T. T. (2007). A component based noise correction method (CompCor) for BOLD and perfusion based fMRI. *NeuroImage, 37*(1), 90–101.

Ben-Shachar, M., Dougherty, R. F., Deutsch, G. K., & Wandell, B. A. (2011). The development of cortical sensitivity to visual word forms. *Journal of Cognitive Neuroscience, 23*(9), 2387–2399.

Berlin, R. (1887). *Eine besondere Art der Wortblindheit (Dyslexie)* (1. Auflage). Wiesbaden: Bergmann.

Bishop, E. G., Cherny, S. S., Corley, R., Plomin, R., DeFries, J. C., & Hewitt, J. K. (2003). Development genetic analysis of general cognitive ability from 1 to 12 years in a sample of adoptees, biological siblings, and twins. *Intelligence, 31*(1), 31–49.

Biswal, B., Zerrin Yetkin, F., Haughton, V. M., & Hyde, J. S. (1995). Functional connectivity in the motor cortex of resting human brain using echo-planar mri. *Magnetic Resonance in Medicine, 34*(4), 537–541.

Blanton, R. E., Levitt, J. G., Thompson, P. M., Narr, K. L., Capetillo-Cunliffe, L., Nobel, A., ... Toga, A. W. (2001). Mapping cortical asymmetry and complexity patterns in normal children. *Psychiatry Research: Neuroimaging, 107*(1), 29–43.

Bloch, F., Hansen, W. W., & Packard, M. (1946). Nuclear Induction. *Physical Review, 69*(3-4), 127–127.

Boets, B., Op de Beeck, H., Vandermosten, M., Scott, S. K., Gillebert, C. R., Mantini, D., ... Ghesquière, P. (2013). Intact but less accessible phonetic representations in adults with dyslexia. *Science, 342*(6163), 1251–1254.

Booth, J. R., Burman, D. D., Meyer, J. R., Gitelman, D. R., Parrish, T. B., & Mesulam, M. M. (2004). Development of brain mechanisms for processing orthographic and phonologic representations. *Journal of Cognitive Neuroscience, 16*(7), 1234–1249.

Borowsky, R., Cummine, J., Owen, W. J., Friesen, C. K., Shih, F., & Sarty, G. E. (2006). FMRI of ventral and dorsal processing streams in basic reading processes: Insular sensitivity to phonology. *Brain Topography, 18*(4), 233–239.

Bosse, M.-L., Tainturier, M.-J., & Valdois, S. (2007). Developmental dyslexia: The visual attention span deficit hypothesis. *Cognition, 104*(2), 198–230.

Brem, S., Bach, S., Kucian, K., Kujala, J. V., Guttorm, T. K., Martin, E., ... Richardson, U. (2010). Brain sensitivity to print emerges when children learn letter–speech sound correspondences. *Proceedings of the National Academy of Sciences of the United States of America, 107*(17), 7939–7944.

Bremner, J. G., Slater, A. M., Hayes, R. A., Mason, U. C., Murphy, C., Spring, J., ... Johnson, S. P. (2017). Young infants' visual fixation patterns in addition and subtraction tasks support an object tracking account. *Journal of Experimental Child Psychology, 162*, 199–208.

Breukelaar, I. A., Antees, C., Grieve, S. M., Foster, S. L., Gomes, L., Williams, L. M., & Korgaonkar, M. S. (2017). Cognitive control network anatomy correlates with neurocognitive behavior: A longitudinal study. *Human Brain Mapping*, *38*(2), 631–643.

Brodmann, K. (1909). *Vergleichende Lokalisationslehre der Grosshirnrinde in ihren Prinzipien dargestellt auf Grund des Zellenbaues*. Leipzig: Barth.

Brody, B. A., Kinney, H. C., Kloman, A. S., & Gilles, F. H. (1987). Sequence of central nervous system myelination in human infancy. I. An autopsy study of myelination. *Journal of Neuropathology & Experimental Neurology*, *46*(3), 283–301.

Brown, M., Askew, M., Rhodes, V., Denvir, H., Ranson, E., & Wiliam, D. (2003). Characterising individual and cohort progression in learning numeracy: Results from the Leverhulme 5-year longitudinal study. (pp. 21–25). Chicago.

Brown, T. T., & Jernigan, T. L. (2012). Brain development during the preschool years. *Neuropsychology Review*, *22*(4), 313–333.

Brown, T. T., Kuperman, J., Chung, Y., Erhart, M., McCabe, C., Hagler Jr., D., … Dale, A. (2012). Neuroanatomical assessment of biological maturity. *Current Biology*, *22*(18), 1693–1698.

Buchanan, C. R., Pernet, C. R., Gorgolewski, K. J., Storkey, A. J., & Bastin, M. E. (2014). Test–retest reliability of structural brain networks from diffusion MRI. *NeuroImage*, *86*, 231–243.

Budday, S., Raybaud, C., & Kuhl, E. (2014). A mechanical model predicts morphological abnormalities in the developing human brain. *Scientific Reports*, *4*(1), 4:5644.

Budday, S., & Steinmann, P. (2018). On the influence of inhomogeneous stiffness and growth on mechanical instabilities in the developing brain. *International Journal of Solids and Structures*, *132*, 31–41.

Budday, S., Steinmann, P., & Kuhl, E. (2015a). Physical biology of human brain development. *Frontiers in Cellular Neuroscience*, *9*, 257.

Budday, S., Steinmann, P., & Kuhl, E. (2015b). Secondary instabilities modulate cortical complexity in the mammalian brain. *Philosophical Magazine*, *95*(28-30), 3244–3256.

Burton, D. M. (2011). *The history of mathematics: An introduction* (7th ed.). New York, NY, US: McGraw-Hill.

Burton, M. W., LoCasto, P. C., Krebs-Noble, D., & Gullapalli, R. P. (2005). A systematic investigation of the functional neuroanatomy of auditory and visual phonological processing. *NeuroImage*, *26*(3), 647–661.

Butterworth, B., & Kovas, Y. (2013). Understanding neurocognitive developmental disorders can improve education for all. *Science*, *340*(6130), 300–305.

Cafiero, R., Brauer, J., Anwander, A., & Friederici, A. D. (2018). The concurrence of cortical surface area expansion and white matter myelination in human brain development. *Cerebral Cortex*, *29*(2), 827–837.

Cantlon, J. F., Brannon, E. M., Carter, E. J., & Pelphrey, K. A. (2006). Functional imaging of numerical processing in adults and 4-y-old children. *PLOS Biology*, *4*(5), e125.

Cao, Q.-J., Zang, Y.-F., Sun, L., Sui, M., Long, X.-Y., Zou, Q.-H., & Wang, Y.-F. (2006). Abnormal neural activity in children with attention deficit hyperactivity disorder: A resting–state functional magnetic resonance imaging study. *NeuroReport*, *17*(10), 1033–1036.

Carneiro, P., Meghir, C., & Parey, M. (2013). Maternal education, home environments, and the development of children and adolescents. *Journal of the European Economic Association*, *11*(S1), 123–160.

Carreiras, M., Armstrong, B. C., Perea, M., & Frost, R. (2014). The what, when, where, and how of visual word recognition. *Trends in Cognitive Sciences*, *18*(2), 90–98.

Carreiras, M., Seghier, M. L., Baquero, S., Estévez, A., Lozano, A., Devlin, J. T., & Price, C. J. (2009). An anatomical signature for literacy. *Nature*, *461*(7266), 983–986.

Casey, B. J., Tottenham, N., Liston, C., & Durston, S. (2005). Imaging the developing brain: What have we learned about cognitive development? *Trends in Cognitive Sciences*, *9*(3), 104–110.

Centanni, T. M., Booker, A. M., Sloan, A. M., Chen, F., Maher, B. J., Carraway, R. S., . . . Kilgard, M. P. (2014). Knockdown of the dyslexia-associated gene Kiaa0319 impairs temporal responses to speech stimuli in rat primary auditory cortex. *Cerebral Cortex*, *24*(7), 1753–1766.

Centanni, T. M., Chen, F., Booker, A. M., Engineer, C. T., Sloan, A. M., Rennaker, R. L., . . . Kilgard, M. P. (2014). Speech sound processing deficits and training-induced neural plasticity in rats with dyslexia gene knockdown. *PLOS ONE*, *9*(5), e98439.

Chai, X. J., Castañón, A. N., Öngür, D., & Whitfield-Gabrieli, S. (2012). Anticorrelations in resting state networks without global signal regression. *NeuroImage*, *59*(2), 1420–1428.

Cho, S., Ryali, S., Geary, D. C., & Menon, V. (2011). How does a child solve 7 + 8? Decoding brain activity patterns associated with counting and retrieval strategies. *Developmental Science*, *14*(5), 989–1001.

Clark, K. A., Helland, T., Specht, K., Narr, K. L., Manis, F. R., Toga, A. W., & Hugdahl, K. (2014). Neuroanatomical precursors of dyslexia identified from pre-reading through to age 11. *Brain*, *137*(12), 3136–3141.

Cockcroft, W. H. (1982). *Mathematics counts*. HM Stationery Office. London.

Cohen, L., Dehaene, S., Naccache, L., Lehéricy, S., Dehaene-Lambertz, G., Hénaff, M.-A., & Michel, F. (2000). The visual word form areaSpatial and temporal characterization of an initial stage of reading in normal subjects and posterior split-brain patients. *Brain*, *123*(2), 291–307.

Coltheart, M., Rastle, K., Perry, C., Langdon, R., & Ziegler, J. (2001). DRC: A dual route cascaded model of visual word recognition and reading aloud. *Psychological Review*, *108*(1), 204–256.

Corbetta, M., Kincade, J. M., Ollinger, J. M., McAvoy, M. P., & Shulman, G. L. (2000). Voluntary orienting is dissociated from target detection in human posterior parietal cortex. *Nature Neuroscience*, *3*(3), 292–297.

Cox, R. W. (1996). AFNI: Software for analysis and visualization of functional magnetic resonance neuroimages. *Computers and Biomedical Research, 29*(3), 162–173.

Cox, R. W., & Hyde, J. S. (1997). Software tools for analysis and visualization of fMRI data. *NMR in Biomedicine, 10*(4-5), 171–178.

Cragg, B. G. (1975). The density of synapses and neurons in normal, mentally defective ageing human brains. *Brain, 98*(1), 81–90.

Dahnke, R., & Gaser, C. (2018). Surface and shape analysis. In G. Spalletta, F. Piras, & T. Gili (Eds.), *Brain morphometry* (pp. 51–73). New York, NY, US: Humana Press.

Dahnke, R., Yotter, R. A., & Gaser, C. (2013). Cortical thickness and central surface estimation. *NeuroImage, 65*, 336–348.

Dale, A. M., Fischl, B., & Sereno, M. I. (1999). Cortical surface-based analysis. I. Segmentation and surface reconstruction. *NeuroImage, 9*(2), 179–194.

Dale, B. M., Brown, M. A., & Semelka, R. C. (2015). *MRI: Basic principles and applications* (5th ed.). John Wiley & Sons Ltd.

Davis, O. S. P., Band, G., Pirinen, M., Haworth, C. M. A., Meaburn, E. L., Kovas, Y., . . . Spencer, C. C. A. (2014). The correlation between reading and mathematics ability at age twelve has a substantial genetic component. *Nature Communications, 5*, 4204.

De Smedt, B., Holloway, I. D., & Ansari, D. (2011). Effects of problem size and arithmetic operation on brain activation during calculation in children with varying levels of arithmetical fluency. *NeuroImage*. Special Issue: Educational Neuroscience, 57(3), 771–781.

De Smedt, B., Taylor, J., Archibald, L., & Ansari, D. (2010). How is phonological processing related to individual differences in children's arithmetic skills? *Developmental Science, 13*(3), 508–520.

de Haan, M., Pascalis, O., & Johnson, M. H. (2002). Specialization of neural mechanisms underlying face recognition in human infants. *Journal of Cognitive Neuroscience, 14*(2), 199–209.

de Schotten, T. M., Cohen, L., Amemiya, E., Braga, L. W., & Dehaene, S. (2014). Learning to read improves the structure of the arcuate fasciculus. *Cerebral Cortex, 24*(4), 989–995.

Dehaene, S. (2011). *The number sense: How the mind creates mathematics, revised and updated edition*. Oxford University Press, USA.

Dehaene, S., Bossini, S., & Giraux, P. (1993). The mental representation of parity and number magnitude. *Journal of Experimental Psychology: General, 122*(3), 371–396.

Dehaene, S., Pegado, F., Braga, L. W., Ventura, P., Filho, G. N., Jobert, A., . . . Cohen, L. (2010). How learning to read changes the cortical networks for vision and language. *Science, 330*(6009), 1359–1364.

Dehaene, S., Piazza, M., Pinel, P., & Cohen, L. (2003). Three parietal circuits for number processing. *Cognitive Neuropsychology, 20*(3-6), 487–506.

Deichmann, R. (2016). Principles of MRI and functional MRI. In M. Filippi (Ed.), *fMRI Techniques and Protocols* (2nd ed., pp. 3–28). New York, NY: Springer New York.

Devine, A., Soltész, F., Nobes, A., Goswami, U., & Szűcs, D. (2013). Gender differences in developmental dyscalculia depend on diagnostic criteria. *Learning and Instruction*, *27*, 31–39.

Devlin, J. T., Sillery, E., Hall, D. A., Hobden, P., Behrens, T. E. J., Nunes, R. G., … Johansen-Berg, H. (2006). Reliable identification of the auditory thalamus using multi-modal structural analyses. *NeuroImage*, *30*(4), 1112–1120.

Díaz, B., Hintz, F., Kiebel, S. J., & von Kriegstein, K. (2012). Dysfunction of the auditory thalamus in developmental dyslexia. *Proceedings of the National Academy of Sciences of the United States of America*, *109*(34), 13841–13846.

Diedrichsen, J. (2006). A spatially unbiased atlas template of the human cerebellum. *NeuroImage*, *33*(1), 127–138.

Diedrichsen, J., Balsters, J. H., Flavell, J., Cussans, E., & Ramnani, N. (2009). A probabilistic MR atlas of the human cerebellum. *NeuroImage*, *46*(1), 39–46.

Dirks, E., Spyer, G., van Lieshout, E. C. D. M., & de Sonneville, L. (2008). Prevalence of combined reading and arithmetic disabilities. *Journal of Learning Disabilities*, *41*(5), 460–473.

Doria, V., Beckmann, C. F., Arichi, T., Merchant, N., Groppo, M., Turkheimer, F. E., … Edwards, A. D. (2010). Emergence of resting state networks in the preterm human brain. *Proceedings of the National Academy of Sciences of the United States of America*, *107*(46), 20015–20020.

Draganski, B., Gaser, C., Busch, V., Schuierer, G., Bogdahn, U., & May, A. (2004). Changes in grey matter induced by training. *Nature*, *427*(6972), 311–312.

Draganski, B., Gaser, C., Kempermann, G., Kuhn, H. G., Winkler, J., Büchel, C., & May, A. (2006). Temporal and spatial dynamics of brain structure changes during extensive learning. *Journal of Neuroscience*, *26*(23), 6314–6317.

Ducharme, S., Albaugh, M. D., Nguyen, T.-V., Hudziak, J. J., Mateos-Pérez, J. M., Labbe, A., … Karama, S. (2016). Trajectories of cortical thickness maturation in normal brain development — The importance of quality control procedures. *NeuroImage*, *125*, 267–279.

Dufor, O., Serniclaes, W., Sprenger-Charolles, L., & Démonet, J.-F. (2009). Left premotor cortex and allophonic speech perception in dyslexia: A PET study. *NeuroImage*, *46*(1), 241–248.

Duncan, G. J., Dowsett, C. J., Claessens, A., Magnuson, K., Huston, A. C., Klebanov, P., … Japel, C. (2007). School readiness and later achievement. *Developmental Psychology*, *43*(6), 1428–1446.

Durand, M., Hulme, C., Larkin, R., & Snowling, M. J. (2005). The cognitive foundations of reading and arithmetic skills in 7- to 10-year-olds. *Journal of Experimental Child Psychology*, *91*(2), 113–136.

Durston, S., Davidson, M. C., Tottenham, N., Galvan, A., Spicer, J., Fossella, J. A., & Casey, B. J. (2006). A shift from diffuse to focal cortical activity with development. *Developmental Science*, *9*(1), 1–8.

Eckert, M. A., Leonard, C. M., Richards, T. L., Aylward, E., Thomson, J., & Berninger, V. (2003). Anatomical correlates of dyslexia: Frontal and cerebellar findings. *Brain*, *126*(2), 482–494.

Eckert, M. A., Leonard, C. M., Wilke, M., Eckert, M., Richards, T., Richards, A., & Berninger, V. (2005). Anatomical signatures of dyslexia in children: Unique information from manual and voxel based morphometry brain measures. *Cortex*, *41*(3), 304–315.

Eden, G. F., VanMeter, J. W., Rumsey, J. M., Maisog, J. M., Woods, R. P., & Zeffiro, T. A. (1996). Abnormal processing of visual motion in dyslexia revealed by functional brain imaging. *Nature*, *382*(6586), 66–69.

Egorova, N., Veldsman, M., Cumming, T., & Brodtmann, A. (2017). Fractional amplitude of low-frequency fluctuations (fALFF) in post-stroke depression. *NeuroImage: Clinical*, *16*, 116–124.

Elbeheri, G., Everatt, J., & Al Malki, M. (2009). The incidence of dyslexia among young offenders in Kuwait. *Dyslexia*, *15*(2), 86–104.

Elster, A. D. (1993). Gradient-echo MR imaging: Techniques and acronyms. *Radiology*, *186*(1), 1–8.

Ester, E., Sprague, T., & Serences, J. (2015). Parietal and frontal cortex encode stimulus-specific mnemonic representations during visual working memory. *Neuron*, *87*(4), 893–905.

Evans, T. M., Kochalka, J., Ngoon, T. J., Wu, S. S., Qin, S., Battista, C., & Menon, V. (2015). Brain structural integrity and intrinsic functional connectivity forecast 6 year longitudinal growth in children's numerical abilities. *The Journal of Neuroscience*, *35*(33), 11743–11750.

Facoetti, A., Lorusso, M. L., Paganoni, P., Cattaneo, C., Galli, R., & Mascetti, G. G. (2003). The time course of attentional focusing in dyslexic and normally reading children. *Brain and Cognition*, *53*(2), 181–184.

Facoetti, A., Zorzi, M., Cestnick, L., Lorusso, M. L., Molteni, M., Paganoni, P., ... Mascetti, G. G. (2006). The relationship between visuo-spatial attention and nonword reading in developmental dyslexia. *Cognitive Neuropsychology*, *23*(6), 841–855.

Fawcett, A. J., & Nicolson, R. I. (1999). Performance of dyslexic children on cerebellar and cognitive tests. *Journal of Motor Behavior*, *31*(1), 68–78.

Fawcett, A. J., Nicolson, R. I., & Dean, P. (1996). Impaired performance of children with dyslexia on a range of cerebellar tasks. *Annals of Dyslexia*, *46*(1), 259–283.

Feigenson, L., Carey, S., & Hauser, M. (2002). The Representations Underlying Infants' Choice of More: Object Files Versus Analog Magnitudes. *Psychological Science*, *13*(2), 150–156.

Feigenson, L., Dehaene, S., & Spelke, E. S. (2004). Core systems of number. *Trends in Cognitive Sciences*, *8*(7), 307–314.

Fields, R. D., Araque, A., Johansen-Berg, H., Lim, S.-S., Lynch, G., Nave, K.-A., ... Wake, H. (2014). Glial biology in learning and cognition. *The Neuroscientist*, *20*(5), 426–431.

Finch, A. J., Nicolson, R. I., & Fawcett, A. J. (2002). Evidence for a neuroanatomical difference within the olivo-cerebellar pathway of adults with dyslexia. *Cortex*, *38*(4), 529–539.

Fischl, B. (2012). FreeSurfer. *NeuroImage*, *62*(2), 774–781.

Fischl, B., Sereno, M. I., & Dale, A. M. (1999). Cortical surface-based analysis. II: Inflation, flattening, and a surface-based coordinate system. *NeuroImage, 9*(2), 195–207.

Fjell, A. M., Grydeland, H., Krogsrud, S. K., Amlien, I., Rohani, D. A., Ferschmann, L., . . . Walhovd, K. B. (2015). Development and aging of cortical thickness correspond to genetic organization patterns. *Proceedings of the National Academy of Sciences of the United States of America, 112*(50), 15462–15467.

Fletcher, J. M., & Loveland, K. A. (1986). Neuropsychology of arithmetic disabilities in children. *Focus on Learning Problems in Mathematics, 8*(2), 23–40.

FMRIB Analysis Group. (2015). FSL. Oxford, UK. Retrieved from https://fsl.fmrib.ox.ac.uk/fsl/fslwiki/

Fonov, V. S., Evans, A. C., Botteron, K., Almli, C. R., McKinstry, R. C., & Collins, D. L. (2011). Unbiased average age-appropriate atlases for pediatric studies. *NeuroImage, 54*(1), 313–327.

Fonov, V. S., Evans, A. C., McKinstry, R. C., Almli, C. R., & Collins, D. L. (2009). Unbiased nonlinear average age-appropriate brain templates from birth to adulthood. *NeuroImage, Supplement 1*(47), S102.

Fox, M. D., Snyder, A. Z., Vincent, J. L., Corbetta, M., & Raichle, M. E. (2005). The human brain is intrinsically organized into dynamic, anticorrelated functional networks. *Proceedings of the National Academy of Sciences of the United States of America, 102*(27), 9673–9678.

Foxton, J. M., Talcott, J. B., Witton, C., Brace, H., McIntyre, F., & Griffiths, T. D. (2003). Reading skills are related to global, but not local, acoustic pattern perception. *Nature Neuroscience, 6*(4), 343–344.

Fransson, P., Skiöld, B., Horsch, S., Nordell, A., Blennow, M., Lagercrantz, H., & Åden, U. (2007). Resting-state networks in the infant brain. *Proceedings of the National Academy of Sciences of the United States of America, 104*(39), 15531–15536.

FreeSurfer. (2014). Retrieved from http://surfer.nmr.mgh.harvard.edu/

Friederici, A. D. (2018). The neural basis for human syntax: Broca's area and beyond. *Current Opinion in Behavioral Sciences*. The Evolution of Language, *21*, 88–92.

Friston, K. J., Ashburner, J. T., Kiebel, S. J., Nichols, T. E., & Penny, W. D. (Eds.). (2007). *Statistical parametric mapping: The analysis of functional brain images*. Elsevier.

Fryer, S. L., Roach, B. J., Ford, J. M., Turner, J. A., van Erp, T. G. M., Voyvodic, J., . . . Mathalon, D. H. (2015). Relating Intrinsic Low-Frequency BOLD Cortical Oscillations to Cognition in Schizophrenia. *Neuropsychopharmacology, 40*(12), 2705–2714.

Galaburda, A. M., & Kemper, T. L. (1979). Cytoarchitectonic abnormalities in developmental dyslexia: A case study. *Annals of Neurology, 6*(2), 94–100.

Galaburda, A. M., LoTurco, J., Ramus, F., Fitch, R. H., & Rosen, G. D. (2006). From genes to behavior in developmental dyslexia. *Nature Neuroscience, 9*(10), 1213–1217.

Galaburda, A. M., Menard, M. T., & Rosen, G. D. (1994). Evidence for aberrant auditory anatomy in developmental dyslexia. *Proceedings of the National Academy of Sciences of the United States of America, 91*(17), 8010–8013.

Galaburda, A. M., Sherman, G. F., Rosen, G. D., Aboitiz, F., & Geschwind, N. (1985). Developmental dyslexia: Four consecutive patients with cortical anomalies. *Annals of Neurology, 18*(2), 222–233.

Gao, W., Lin, W., Chen, Y., Gerig, G., Smith, J. K., Jewells, V., & Gilmore, J. H. (2009). Temporal and spatial development of axonal maturation and myelination of white matter in the developing brain. *American Journal of Neuroradiology, 30*(2), 290–296.

Gaser, C., & Dahnke, R. (2017). Computational Anatomy Toolbox. Jena, Germany: Structural Brain Mapping Group. Retrieved from http://www.neuro.uni-jena.de/cat/index.html

Geary, D. C. (2011). Cognitive predictors of achievement growth in mathematics: A five year longitudinal study. *Developmental psychology, 47*(6), 1539–1552.

Gilmore, J. H., Knickmeyer, R. C., & Gao, W. (2018). Imaging structural and functional brain development in early childhood. *Nature Reviews Neuroscience, 19*(3), 123–137.

Giraud, A.-L., & Poeppel, D. (2012). Cortical oscillations and speech processing: Emerging computational principles and operations. *Nature Neuroscience, 15*(4), 511–517.

Glasser, M. F., Coalson, T. S., Robinson, E. C., Hacker, C. D., Harwell, J., Yacoub, E., … Van Essen, D. C. (2016). A multi-modal parcellation of human cerebral cortex. *Nature, 536*(7615), 171–178.

Glezer, L. S., Jiang, X., & Riesenhuber, M. (2009). Evidence for highly selective neuronal tuning to whole words in the "visual word form area". *Neuron, 62*(2), 199–204.

Goswami, U. (2015). Sensory theories of developmental dyslexia: Three challenges for research. *Nature Reviews Neuroscience, 16*(1), 43–54.

Goswami, U., Thomson, J., Richardson, U., Stainthorp, R., Hughes, D., Rosen, S., & Scott, S. K. (2002). Amplitude envelope onsets and developmental dyslexia: A new hypothesis. *Proceedings of the National Academy of Sciences of the United States of America, 99*(16), 10911–10916.

Grabner, R. H., Ansari, D., Reishofer, G., Stern, E., Ebner, F., & Neuper, C. (2007). Individual differences in mathematical competence predict parietal brain activation during mental calculation. *NeuroImage, 38*(2), 346–356.

Grasby, K. L., Coventry, W. L., Byrne, B., Olson, R. K., & Medland, S. E. (2016). Genetic and environmental influences on literacy and numeracy performance in australian school children in grades 3, 5, 7, and 9. *Behavior Genetics, 46*(5), 627–648.

Gross, J. (2009). *The Long Term Costs of Literacy Difficulties. 2nd edition.* KPMG Foundation.

Grosse Wiesmann, C., Schreiber, J., Singer, T., Steinbeis, N., & Friederici, A. D. (2017). White matter maturation is associated with the emergence of Theory of Mind in early childhood. *Nature Communications, 8*, 14692.

Grotheer, M., Ambrus, G. G., & Kovács, G. (2016). Causal evidence of the involvement of the number form area in the visual detection of numbers and letters. *NeuroImage, 132*, 314–319.

Grotheer, M., Jeska, B., & Grill-Spector, K. (2018). A preference for mathematical processing outweighs the selectivity for Arabic numbers in the inferior temporal gyrus. *NeuroImage*, *175*, 188–200.

Haffner, J., Baro, K., Parzer, P., & Resch, F. (2005). *Heidelberger Rechentest (HRT 1-4)*. Göttingen: Hogrefe.

Haft, S. L., Duong, P. H., Ho, T. C., Hendren, R. L., & Hoeft, F. (2018). Anxiety and Attentional Bias in Children with Specific Learning Disorders. *Journal of Abnormal Child Psychology*, 1–11.

Halliday, L. F., & Bishop, D. V. M. (2006). Is poor frequency modulation detection linked to literacy problems? A comparison of specific reading disability and mild to moderate sensorineural hearing loss. *Brain and Language, 97*(2), 200–213.

Hämäläinen, J. A., Leppänen, P. H. T., Eklund, K., Thomson, J. M., Richardson, U., Guttorm, T. K., . . . Lyytinen, H. (2009). Common variance in amplitude envelope perception tasks and their impact on phoneme duration perception and reading and spelling in Finnish children with reading disabilities. *Applied Psycholinguistics, 30*(3), 511–530.

Hampson, M., Driesen, N. R., Roth, J. K., Gore, J. C., & Constable, R. T. (2010). Functional connectivity between task-positive and task-negative brain areas and its relation to working memory performance. *Magnetic Resonance Imaging, 28*(8), 1051–1057.

Hampson, M., Driesen, N. R., Skudlarski, P., Gore, J. C., & Constable, R. T. (2006). Brain connectivity related to working memory performance. *Journal of Neuroscience, 26*(51), 13338–13343.

Harm, M. W., & Seidenberg, M. S. (1999). Phonology, reading acquisition, and dyslexia: Insights from connectionist models. *Psychological Review, 106*(3), 491–528.

Hart, S. A., Petrill, S. A., Thompson, L. A., & Plomin, R. (2009). The ABCs of math: A genetic analysis of mathematics and its links with reading ability and general cognitive ability. *Journal of educational psychology, 101*(2), 388.

Hasegawa, M., Houdou, S., Mito, T., Takashima, S., Asanuma, K., & Ohno, T. (1992). Development of myelination in the human fetal and infant cerebrum: A myelin basic protein immunohistochemical study. *Brain and Development, 14*(1), 1–6.

Haworth, C. M. A., Kovas, Y., Harlaar, N., Hayiou-Thomas, M. E., Petrill, S. A., Dale, P. S., & Plomin, R. (2009). Generalist genes and learning disabilities: A multivariate genetic analysis of low performance in reading, mathematics, language and general cognitive ability in a sample of 8000 12-year-old twins. *Journal of Child Psychology and Psychiatry, 50*(10), 1318–1325.

Hecht, S. A., Torgesen, J. K., Wagner, R. K., & Rashotte, C. A. (2001). The relations between phonological processing abilities and emerging individual differences in mathematical computation skills: A longitudinal study from second to fifth grades. *Journal of Experimental Child Psychology, 79*(2), 192–227.

Heim, S. [Sabine], Freeman Jr., R. B., Eulitz, C., & Elbert, T. (2001). Auditory temporal processing deficit in dyslexia is associated with enhanced sensitivity in the visual modality. *NeuroReport, 12*(3), 507–510.

Heim, S. [Stefan], Tschierse, J., Amunts, K., Wilms, M., Vossel, S., Willmes, K., ... Huber, W. (2008). Cognitive subtypes of dyslexia. *Acta neurobiologiae experimentalis*, *68*, 73–82.

Helenius, P., Uutela, K., & Hari, R. (1999). Auditory stream segregation in dyslexic adults. *Brain*, *122*(5), 907–913.

Herman, A. E., Galaburda, A. M., Fitch, R. H., Carter, A. R., & Rosen, G. D. (1997). Cerebral microgyria, thalamic cell size and auditory temporal processing in male and female rats. *Cerebral Cortex*, *7*(5), 453–464.

Hermes, D., Rangarajan, V., Foster, B. L., King, J.-R., Kasikci, I., Miller, K. J., & Parvizi, J. (2017). Electrophysiological responses in the ventral temporal cortex during reading of numerals and calculation. *Cerebral Cortex*, *27*(1), 567–575.

Hill, N. I., Bailey, P. J., Griffiths, Y. M., & Snowling, M. J. (1999). Frequency acuity and binaural masking release in dyslexic listeners. *The Journal of the Acoustical Society of America*, *106*(6), L53–L58.

Hoeft, F., Hernandez, A., McMillon, G., Taylor-Hill, H., Martindale, J. L., Keller, T. A., ... Gabrieli, J. D. E. (2007). Functional and morphometric brain dissociation between dyslexia and reading ability. *Proceedings of the National Academy of Sciences of the United States of America*, *104*(10), 4234–4239.

Hoeft, F., McCandliss, B. D., Black, J. M., Gantman, A., Zakerani, N., Hulme, C., ... Gabrieli, J. D. E. (2011). Neural systems predicting long-term outcome in dyslexia. *Proceedings of the National Academy of Sciences of the United States of America*, *108*(1), 361–366.

Hoffstaedter, F., Grefkes, C., Roski, C., Caspers, S., Zilles, K., & Eickhoff, S. B. (2015). Age-related decrease of functional connectivity additional to gray matter atrophy in a network for movement initiation. *Brain Structure and Function*, *220*(2), 999–1012.

Hofman, M. A. (2012). Design principles of the human brain. In Hofman, Michel A. & Falk, D. (Eds.), *Progress in Brain Research* (Vol. 195, pp. 373–390). Elsevier.

Hoptman, M. J., Zuo, X.-N., Butler, P. D., Javitt, D. C., D'Angelo, D., Mauro, C. J., & Milham, M. P. (2010). Amplitude of low-frequency oscillations in schizophrenia: A resting state fMRI study. *Schizophrenia Research*, *117*(1), 13.

Hornickel, J., & Kraus, N. (2013). Unstable representation of sound: A biological marker of dyslexia. *Journal of Neuroscience*, *33*(8), 3500–3504.

Howard Jr., J. H., Howard, D. V., Japikse, K. C., & Eden, G. F. (2005). Dyslexics are impaired on implicit higher-order sequence learning, but not on implicit spatial context learning. *Neuropsychologia*, *44*(7), 1131–1144.

Hu, W., Lee, H. L., Zhang, Q., Liu, T., Geng, L. B., Seghier, M. L., ... Price, C. J. (2010). Developmental dyslexia in Chinese and English populations: Dissociating the effect of dyslexia from language differences. *Brain*, *133*(6), 1694–1706.

Huettig, F., Lachmann, T., Reis, A., & Petersson, K. M. (2018). Distinguishing cause from effect – many deficits associated with developmental dyslexia may be a consequence of reduced and suboptimal reading experience. *Language, Cognition and Neuroscience*, *33*(3), 333–350.

Huttenlocher, P. R., & Dabholkar, A. S. (1997). Regional differences in synaptogenesis in human cerebral cortex. *Journal of Comparative Neurology*, *387*(2), 167–178.

Im, K., Raschle, N. M., Smith, S. A., Ellen Grant, P., & Gaab, N. (2016). Atypical sulcal pattern in children with developmental dyslexia and at-risk kindergarteners. *Cerebral Cortex*, *26*(3), 1138–1148.

Innocenti, G. M., & Price, D. J. (2005). Exuberance in the development of cortical networks. *Nature Reviews Neuroscience*, *6*(12), 955–965.

Jackson, N. E., & Butterfield, E. C. (1989). Reading-level-match designs: Myths and realities. *Journal of Reading Behavior*, *21*(4), 387–412.

Jansen, H., Mannhaupt, G., Marx, H., & Skowronek, H. (1999). *Bielefelder Screening zur Früherkennung von Lese-Rechtschreibschwierigkeiten (BISC)*. Göttingen: Hogrefe.

Jednoróg, K., Gawron, N., Marchewka, A., Heim, S., & Grabowska, A. (2014). Cognitive subtypes of dyslexia are characterized by distinct patterns of grey matter volume. *Brain Structure and Function*, *219*(5), 1697–1707.

Jenkinson, M., Bannister, P., Brady, M., & Smith, S. (2002). Improved optimization for the robust and accurate linear registration and motion correction of brain images. *NeuroImage*, *17*(2), 825–841.

Jenkinson, M., Beckmann, C. F., Behrens, T. E. J., Woolrich, M. W., & Smith, S. M. (2012). FSL. *NeuroImage*. 20 YEARS OF fMRI, *62*(2), 782–790.

Jenkinson, M., & Smith, S. (2001). A global optimisation method for robust affine registration of brain images. *Medical Image Analysis*, *5*(2), 143–156.

Jessell, T. M., & Sanes, J. R. (2013). Differentiation and survival of nerve cells. In E. R. Kandel, J. H. Schwartz, T. M. Jessell, S. A. Siegelbaum, & A. J. Hudspeth (Eds.), *Principles of neural science* (pp. 1187–1208). 5. New York: McGraw Hill Medical.

Jiang, L., Xu, T., He, Y., Hou, X.-H., Wang, J., Cao, X.-Y., ... Zuo, X.-N. (2015). Toward neurobiological characterization of functional homogeneity in the human cortex: Regional variation, morphological association and functional covariance network organization. *Brain Structure and Function*, *220*(5), 2485–2507.

Jobard, G., Crivello, F., & Tzourio-Mazoyer, N. (2003). Evaluation of the dual route theory of reading: A metanalysis of 35 neuroimaging studies. *NeuroImage*, *20*(2), 693–712.

Johannes, S., Kussmaul, C. L., Münte, T. F., & Mangun, G. R. (1996). Developmental dyslexia: Passive visual stimulation provides no evidence for a magnocellular processing defect. *Neuropsychologia*, *34*(11), 1123–1127.

Johnson, M. H. (2001). Functional brain development in humans. *Nature Reviews Neuroscience*, *2*(7), 475–483.

Jolles, D., Ashkenazi, S., Kochalka, J., Evans, T. M., Richardson, J., Rosenberg-Lee, M., ... Menon, V. (2016). Parietal hyper-connectivity, aberrant brain organization, and circuit- based biomarkers in children with mathematical disabilities. *Developmental Science*, *19*(4), 613–631.

Jolles, D., Supekar, K., Richardson, J., Tenison, C., Ashkenazi, S., Rosenberg-Lee, M., ... Menon, V. (2016). Reconfiguration of parietal circuits with cognitive tutoring in elementary school children. *Cortex*, *83*, 231–245.

Jones, S. E., Buchbinder, B. R., & Aharon, I. (2000). Three-dimensional mapping of cortical thickness using Laplace's Equation. *Human Brain Mapping*, *11*(1), 12–32.

Kanai, R., & Rees, G. (2011). The structural basis of inter-individual differences in human behaviour and cognition. *Nature Reviews Neuroscience, 12*(4), 231–242.

Kandel, E. R., Barres, B. A., & Hudspeth, A. J. (2013). Nerve Cells, Neural Circuitry, and Behavior. In E. R. Kandel, J. H. Schwartz, T. M. Jessell, S. A. Siegelbaum, & A. J. Hudspeth (Eds.), *Principles of neural science* (pp. 21–38). 5. New York: McGraw Hill Medical.

Kandel, E. R., & Hudspeth, A. J. (2013). The brain and behavior. In E. R. Kandel, J. H. Schwartz, T. M. Jessell, S. A. Siegelbaum, & A. J. Hudspeth (Eds.), *Principles of neural science* (pp. 5–20). 5. New York: McGraw Hill Medical.

Karni, A., Meyer, G., Rey-Hipolito, C., Jezzard, P., Adams, M. M., Turner, R., & Ungerleider, L. G. (1998). The acquisition of skilled motor performance: Fast and slow experience-driven changes in primary motor cortex. *Proceedings of the National Academy of Sciences of the United States of America, 95*(3), 861–868.

Kaufman, A., Kaufman, N., Melchers, U., & Preuß, U. (2009). *K-ABC: Kaufman Assessment Battery for Children. German Version.* Frankfurt am Main: Pearson Assessment.

Kharitonova, M., Martin, R. E., Gabrieli, J. D. E., & Sheridan, M. A. (2013). Cortical gray-matter thinning is associated with age-related improvements on executive function tasks. *Developmental Cognitive Neuroscience, 6*, 61–71.

Kim, J. S., Singh, V., Lee, J. K., Lerch, J., Ad-Dab'bagh, Y., MacDonald, D., ... Evans, A. C. (2005). Automated 3-D extraction and evaluation of the inner and outer cortical surfaces using a Laplacian map and partial volume effect classification. *NeuroImage, 27*(1), 210–221.

King, W. M., Giess, S. A., & Lombardino, L. J. (2007). Subtyping of children with developmental dyslexia via bootstrap aggregated clustering and the gap statistic: Comparison with the double-deficit hypothesis. *International Journal of Language & Communication Disorders, 42*(1), 77–95.

Kinney, H. C., Brody, B. A., Kloman, A. S., & Gilles, F. H. (1988). Sequence of central nervous system myelination in human infancy. II. Patterns of myelination in autopsied infants. *Journal of Neuropathology & Experimental Neurology, 47*(3), 217–234.

Klassen, R. M., Tze, V. M. C., & Hannok, W. (2013). Internalizing problems of adults with learning disabilities: A meta-analysis. *Journal of Learning Disabilities, 46*(4), 317–327.

Knops, A., Thirion, B., Hubbard, E. M., Michel, V., & Dehaene, S. (2009). Recruitment of an area involved in eye movements during mental arithmetic. *Science, 324*(5934), 1583–1585.

Kovas, Y., Haworth, C. M. A., Dale, P. S., & Plomin, R. (2007). The genetic and environmental origins of learning abilities and disabilities in the early school years. *Monographs of the Society for Research in Child Development, 72*(3), 1–144.

Kovas, Y., Haworth, C. M. A., Harlaar, N., Petrill, S. A., Dale, P. S., & Plomin, R. (2007). Overlap and specificity of genetic and environmental influences on mathematics and reading disability in 10-year-old twins. *Journal of Child Psychology and Psychiatry, 48*(9), 914–922.

Krafnick, A. J., Flowers, D. L., Luetje, M. M., Napoliello, E. M., & Eden, G. F. (2014). An investigation into the origin of anatomical differences in dyslexia. *The Journal of Neuroscience, 34*(3), 901–908.

Kraft, I., Cafiero, R., Schaadt, G., Brauer, J., Neef, N. E., Müller, B., . . . Skeide, M. A. (2015). Cortical differences in preliterate children at familiar risk of dyslexia are similar to those observed in dyslexic readers. *Brain, 138*(9), e378–e378.

Kraft, I., Schreiber, J., Cafiero, R., Metere, R., Schaadt, G., Brauer, J., . . . Skeide, M. A. (2016). Predicting early signs of dyslexia at a preliterate age by combining behavioral assessment with structural MRI. *NeuroImage, 143*, 378–386.

Kronbichler, M., Hutzler, F., & Wimmer, H. (2002). Dyslexia: Verbal impairments in the absence of magnocellular impairments. *NeuroReport, 13*(5), 617–620.

Kußmaul, A. (1877). *Die Störungen der Sprache: Versuch einer Pathologie der Sprache.* Leipzig: F.C.W. Vogel.

la Fougère, C., Grant, S., Kostikov, A., Schirrmacher, R., Gravel, P., Schipper, H. M., . . . Thiel, A. (2011). Where in-vivo imaging meets cytoarchitectonics: The relationship between cortical thickness and neuronal density measured with high-resolution [18f]flumazenil-PET. *NeuroImage, 56*(3), 951–960.

Lachmann, T., & van Leeuwen, C. (2014). Reading as functional coordination: Not recycling but a novel synthesis. *Frontiers in Psychology, 5*, 1046.

Landerl, K., Fussenegger, B., Moll, K., & Willburger, E. (2009). Dyslexia and dyscalculia: Two learning disorders with different cognitive profiles. *Journal of Experimental Child Psychology, 103*(3), 309–324.

Lauterbur, P. C. (1973). Image formation by induced local interactions: Examples employing Nuclear Magnetic Resonance. *Nature, 242*, 190–191.

Le Bihan, D., Mangin, J.-F., Poupon, C., Clark, C. A., Pappata, S., Molko, N., & Chabriat, H. (2001). Diffusion tensor imaging: Concepts and applications. *Journal of Magnetic Resonance Imaging, 13*(4), 534–546.

Lebel, C., & Beaulieu, C. (2011). Longitudinal development of human brain wiring continues from childhood into adulthood. *Journal of Neuroscience, 31*(30), 10937–10947.

Lebel, C., & Deoni, S. (2018). The development of brain white matter microstructure. *NeuroImage, 182*, 207–218.

Lehongre, K., Ramus, F., Villiermet, N., Schwartz, D., & Giraud, A.-L. (2011). Altered low-gamma sampling in auditory cortex accounts for the three main facets of dyslexia. *Neuron, 72*(6), 1080–1090.

Lenroot, R. K., & Giedd, J. N. (2006). Brain development in children and adolescents: Insights from anatomical magnetic resonance imaging. *Neuroscience & Biobehavioral Reviews, 30*(6), 718–729.

Lerch, J. P., & Evans, A. C. (2005). Cortical thickness analysis examined through power analysis and a population simulation. *NeuroImage, 24*(1), 163–173.

Lewis, C., Hitch, G. J., & Walker, P. (1994). The prevalence of specific arithmetic difficulties and specific reading difficulties in 9- to 10-year-old boys and girls. *Journal of Child Psychology and Psychiatry, 35*(2), 283–292.

Li, G., Wang, L., Shi, F., Lyall, A. E., Lin, W., Gilmore, J. H., & Shen, D. (2014). Mapping longitudinal development of local cortical gyrification in infants from birth to 2 years of age. *Journal of Neuroscience, 34*(12), 4228–4238.

Liberman, I. Y., & Shankweiler, D. (1985). Phonology and the problems of learning to read and write. *Remedial and Special Education, 6*(6), 8–17.

Lin, W., Zhu, Q., Gao, W., Chen, Y., Toh, C.-H., Styner, M., . . . Gilmore, J. H. (2008). Functional connectivity MR imaging reveals cortical functional connectivity in the developing brain. *American Journal of Neuroradiology, 29*(10), 1883–1889.

Lipton, J. S., & Spelke, E. S. (2003). Origins of number sense: Large-number discrimination in human infants. *Cognition, 14*(5), 396–401.

Liu, X., Somel, M., Tang, L., Yan, Z., Jiang, X., Guo, S., . . . Khaitovich, P. (2012). Extension of cortical synaptic development distinguishes humans from chimpanzees and macaques. *Genome Research, 22*(4), 611–622.

Livingstone, M. S., & Hubel, D. H. (1988). Segregation of form, color, movement, and depth: Anatomy, physiology, and perception. *Science, 240*(4853), 740–749.

Livingstone, M. S., Rosen, G. D., Drislane, F. W., & Galaburda, A. M. (1991). Physiological and anatomical evidence for a magnocellular defect in developmental dyslexia. *Proceedings of the National Academy of Sciences of the United States of America, 88*, 7943–7947.

Logothetis, N. K., Pauls, J., Augath, M., Trinath, T., & Oeltermann, A. (2001). Neurophysiological investigation of the basis of the fMRI signal. *Nature, 412*(6843), 150–157.

Lohmann, G., von Cramon, D. Y., & Colchester, A. C. F. (2008). Deep sulcal landmarks provide an organizing framework for human cortical folding. *Cerebral Cortex, 18*(6), 1415–1420.

Lovegrove, W. J., Bowling, A., Badcock, D. R., & Blackwood, M. (1980). Specific reading disability: Differences in contrast sensitivity as a function of spatial frequency. *Science, 210*(4468), 439–440.

Lüders, E., Narr, K. L., Bilder, R. M., Szeszko, P. R., Gurbani, M. N., Hamilton, L., . . . Gaser, C. (2008). Mapping the Relationship between Cortical Convolution and Intelligence: Effects of Gender. *Cerebral Cortex, 18*(9), 2019–2026.

Lüders, E., Thompson, P. M., Narr, K. L., Toga, A. W., Jäncke, L., & Gaser, C. (2006). A curvature-based approach to estimate local gyrification on the cortical surface. *NeuroImage, 29*(4), 1224–1230.

Lundberg, I., & Sterner, G. (2006). Reading, arithmetic, and task orientation-How are they related? *Annals of Dyslexia, 56*(2), 361–377.

Lyall, A. E., Shi, F., Geng, X., Woolson, S., Li, G., Wang, L., . . . Gilmore, J. H. (2015). Dynamic development of regional cortical thickness and surface area in early childhood. *Cerebral Cortex, 25*(8), 2204–2212.

Markowitz, E. M., Willemsen, G., Trumbetta, S. L., & Boomsma, D. I. (2005). The etiology of mathematical and reading (dis)ability covariation in a sample of Dutch twins. *Twin Research and Human Genetics, 8*(6), 585–593.

Marques, J. P., Kober, T., Krueger, G., van der Zwaag, W., Van de Moortele, P.-F., & Gruetter, R. (2010). MP2rage, a self bias-field corrected sequence for improved segmentation and T1-mapping at high field. *NeuroImage, 49*(2), 1271–1281.

McDermott, K. B., Petersen, S. E., Watson, J. M., & Ojemann, J. G. (2003). A procedure for identifying regions preferentially activated by attention to semantic and phonological relations using functional magnetic resonance imaging. *Neuropsychologia*, *41*(3), 293–303.

McRobbie, D. W., Moore, E. A., Graves, M. J., & Prince, M. R. (2017). *MRI from Picture to Proton* (3rd ed.). Cambridge University Press.

Mechelli, A., Price, C. J., Friston, K. J., & Ashburner, J. T. (2005). Voxel-based morphometry of the human brain: Methods and applications. *Current Medical Imaging Reviews*, *1*(2), 105–113.

Menon, V. (2010). Developmental cognitive neuroscience of arithmetic: Implications for learning and education. *ZDM: The International Journal on Mathematics Education*, *42*(6), 515–525.

Menon, V. (2015). Arithmetic in the child and adult brain. In R. C. Kadosh & A. Dowker (Eds.), *The Oxford handbook of numerical cognition* (pp. 502–530). Oxford library of psychology. New York, NY, US: Oxford University Press.

Menon, V., Rivera, S. M., White, C. D., Glover, G. H., & Reiss, A. L. (2000). Dissociating prefrontal and parietal cortex activation during arithmetic processing. *NeuroImage*, *12*(4), 357–365.

Mercy, J. A., & Steelman, L. C. (1982). Familial influence on the intellectual attainment of children. *American Sociological Review*, *47*(4), 532–542.

Moll, K., Kunze, S., Neuhoff, N., Bruder, J., & Schulte-Körne, G. (2014). Specific learning disorder: Prevalence and gender differences. *PLOS ONE*, *9*(7), e103537.

Moll, K., & Landerl, K. (2010). *SLRT-II: Lese- und Rechtschreibtest; Weiterentwicklung des Salzburger Lese-und Rechtschreibtests (SLRT)*. Bern: Hans Huber.

Moll, K., Ramus, F., Bartling, J., Bruder, J., Kunze, S., Neuhoff, N., . . . Landerl, K. (2014). Cognitive mechanisms underlying reading and spelling development in five European orthographies. *Learning and Instruction*, *29*, 65–77.

Morgan, W. P. (1896). A case of congenital word blindness. *British Medical Journal*, *2*(1871), 1378–1378.

Mori, S., & Tournier, J.-D. (Eds.). (2014). *Introduction to diffusion tensor imaging*. Elsevier.

Morris, R. D., Stuebing, K. K., Fletcher, J. M., Shaywitz, S. E., Lyon, G. R., Shankweiler, D. P., . . . Shaywitz, B. A. (1998). Subtypes of reading disability: Variability around a phonological core. *Journal of Educational Psychology*, *90*(3), 347–373.

Moyer, R. S., & Landauer, T. K. (1967). Time required for Judgements of Numerical Inequality. *Nature*, *215*(5109), 1519–1520.

Mukamel, R. (2005). Coupling between neuronal firing, field potentials, and fMRI in human auditory cortex. *Science*, *309*(5736), 951–954.

Murphy, K., Birn, R. M., Handwerker, D. A., Jones, T. B., & Bandettini, P. A. (2009). The impact of global signal regression on resting state correlations: Are anti-correlated networks introduced? *NeuroImage*, *44*(3), 893–905.

Murphy, K., & Fox, M. D. (2017). Towards a consensus regarding global signal regression for resting state functional connectivity MRI. *NeuroImage*. Cleaning up the fMRI time series: Mitigating noise with advanced acquisition and correction strategies, *154*, 169–173.

Muschelli, J., Nebel, M. B., Caffo, B. S., Barber, A. D., Pekar, J. J., & Mostofsky, S. H. (2014). Reduction of motion-related artifacts in resting state fMRI using aCompCor. *NeuroImage, 96*, 22–35.

Mussolin, C., De Volder, A., Grandin, C., Schlögel, X., Nassogne, M.-C., & Noël, M.-P. (2009). Neural correlates of symbolic number comparison in developmental dyscalculia. *Journal of Cognitive Neuroscience, 22*(5), 860–874.

Mutlu, A. K., Schneider, M., Debbané, M., Badoud, D., Eliez, S., & Schaer, M. (2013). Sex differences in thickness, and folding developments throughout the cortex. *NeuroImage, 82*, 200–207.

Natu, V. S., Gomez, J., Barnett, M., Jeska, B., Kirilina, E., Jaeger, C., . . . Grill-Spector, K. (2018). Apparent thinning of visual cortex during childhood is associated with myelination, not pruning. *bioRxiv, 368274*.

Nave, K.-A., & Werner, H. B. (2014). Myelination of the nervous system: Mechanisms and functions. *Annual Review of Cell and Developmental Biology, 30*(1), 503–533.

Neniskyte, U., & Gross, C. T. (2017). Errant gardeners: Glial-cell-dependent synaptic pruning and neurodevelopmental disorders. *Nature Reviews Neuroscience, 18*(11), 658–670.

Neville, H. J., Mills, D. L., & Lawson, D. S. (1992). Fractionating language: Different neural subsystems with different sensitive periods. *Cerebral Cortex, 2*(3), 244–258.

Nicolson, R. I., & Fawcett, A. J. (1990). Automaticity: A new framework for dyslexia research? *Cognition, 35*(2), 159–182.

Nicolson, R. I., & Fawcett, A. J. (1994). Comparison of deficits in cognitive and motor skills among children with dyslexia. *Annals of Dyslexia, 44*(1), 147–164.

Nicolson, R. I., & Fawcett, A. J. (2005). Developmental dyslexia, learning and the cerebellum. In W. W. Fleischhacker & D. J. Brooks (Eds.), *Neurodevelopmental Disorders* (pp. 19–36). Vienna: Springer Vienna.

Nicolson, R. I., Fawcett, A. J., Berry, E. L., Jenkins, I. H., Dean, P., & Brooks, D. J. (1999). Association of abnormal cerebellar activation with motor learning difficulties in dyslexic adults. *The Lancet, 353*(9165), 1662–1667.

Nicolson, R. I., Fawcett, A. J., & Dean, P. (2001). Developmental dyslexia: The cerebellar deficit hypothesis. *Trends in Neurosciences, 24*(9), 508–511.

O'Donnell, S., Noseworthy, M. D., Levine, B., & Dennis, M. (2005). Cortical thickness of the frontopolar area in typically developing children and adolescents. *NeuroImage, 24*(4), 948–954.

OECD. (2012). *Closing the gender gap: Act now*. OECD Publishing.

Oldfield, R. (1971). The assessment and analysis of handedness: The Edinburgh inventory. *Neuropsychologia, 9*(1), 97–113.

Paakki, J.-J., Rahko, J., Long, X., Moilanen, I., Tervonen, O., Nikkinen, J., . . . Kiviniemi, V. (2010). Alterations in regional homogeneity of resting-state brain activity in autism spectrum disorders. *Brain Research, 1321*, 169–179.

Park, H.-J., & Friston, K. (2013). Structural and functional brain networks: From connections to cognition. *Science, 342*(6158), 1238411.

Patterson, K., Nestor, P. J., & Rogers, T. T. (2007). Where do you know what you know? The representation of semantic knowledge in the human brain. *Nature Reviews Neuroscience, 8*(12), 976–987.

Paulesu, E., Frith, U., Snowling, M. J., Gallagher, A., Morton, J., Frackowiak, R. S. J., & Frith, C. D. (1996). Is developmental dyslexia a disconnection syndrome? Evidence from PET scanning. *Brain, 119*(1), 143–157.

Pauling, L., & Coryell, C. D. (1936). The magnetic properties and structure of hemoglobin, oxyhemoglobin and carbonmonoxyhemoglobin. *Proceedings of the National Academy of Sciences of the United States of America, 22*, 210–216.

Pennington, B. F., Santerre-Lemmon, L., Rosenberg, J., MacDonald, B., Boada, R., Friend, A., . . . Olson, R. K. (2012). Individual prediction of dyslexia by single versus multiple deficit models. *Journal of Abnormal Psychology, 121*(1), 212–224.

Perry, C., Ziegler, J. C., & Zorzi, M. (2007). Nested incremental modeling in the development of computational theories: The CDP+ model of reading aloud. *Psychological Review, 114*(2), 273–315.

Perry, C., Ziegler, J. C., & Zorzi, M. (2010). Beyond single syllables: Large-scale modeling of reading aloud with the Connectionist Dual Process (CDP++) model. *Cognitive Psychology, 61*(2), 106–151.

Petermann, F., & Petermann, U. (2011). *Wechsler Intelligence Scale for Children: Fourth Edition (WISC-IV). German Version.* Frankfurt am Main: Pearson Assessment.

Peterson, R. L., & Pennington, B. F. (2012). Developmental dyslexia. *The Lancet, 379*(9830), 1997–2007.

Peterson, R. L., Pennington, B. F., Olson, R. K., & Wadsworth, S. J. (2014). Longitudinal stability of phonological and surface subtypes of developmental dyslexia. *Scientific Studies of Reading, 18*(5), 347–362.

Peyrin, C., Lallier, M., Démonet, J.-F., Pernet, C., Baciu, M., Le Bas, J. F., & Valdois, S. (2012). Neural dissociation of phonological and visual attention span disorders in developmental dyslexia: FMRI evidence from two case reports. *Brain and Language, 120*(3), 381–394.

Piazza, M., Izard, V., Pinel, P., Le Bihan, D., & Dehaene, S. (2004). Tuning curves for approximate numerosity in the human intraparietal sulcus. *Neuron, 44*(3), 547–555.

Piazza, M., Mechelli, A., Butterworth, B., & Price, C. J. (2002). Are subitizing and counting implemented as separate or functionally overlapping processes? *NeuroImage, 15*(2), 435–446.

Piazza, M., Mechelli, A., Price, C. J., & Butterworth, B. (2006). Exact and approximate judgements of visual and auditory numerosity: An fMRI study. *Brain Research, 1106*(1), 177–188.

Piazza, M., Pinel, P., Le Bihan, D., & Dehaene, S. (2007). A magnitude code common to numerosities and number symbols in human intraparietal cortex. *Neuron, 53*(2), 293–305.

Plaut, D. C., McClelland, J. L., Seidenberg, M. S., & Patterson, K. E. (1996). Understanding normal and impaired word reading: Computational principles in quasi-regular domains. *Psychological Review, 103*(1), 56–115.

Plomin, R., & Kovas, Y. (2005). Generalist genes and learning disabilities. *Psychological Bulletin, 131*(4), 592–617.

Poldrack, R. A., Wagner, A. D., Prull, M. W., Desmond, J. E., Glover, G. H., & Gabrieli, J. D. E. (1999). Functional specialization for semantic and phonological processing in the left inferior prefrontal cortex. *NeuroImage, 10*(1), 15–35.

Power, A. J., Colling, L. J., Mead, N., Barnes, L., & Goswami, U. (2016). Neural encoding of the speech envelope by children with developmental dyslexia. *Brain and Language, 160*, 1–10.

Power, J. D., Barnes, K. A., Snyder, A. Z., Schlaggar, B. L., & Petersen, S. E. (2012). Spurious but systematic correlations in functional connectivity MRI networks arise from subject motion. *NeuroImage, 59*(3), 2142–2154.

Preston, J. L., Molfese, P. J., Frost, S. J., Mencl, W. E., Fulbright, R. K., Hoeft, F., ... Pugh, K. R. (2016). Print-speech convergence predicts future reading outcomes in early readers. *Psychological Science, 27*(1), 75–84.

Price, C. J. (2012). A review and synthesis of the first 20years of PET and fMRI studies of heard speech, spoken language and reading. *NeuroImage.* 20 YEARS OF fMRI, *62*(2), 816–847.

Price, C. J., & Mechelli, A. (2005). Reading and reading disturbance. *Current Opinion in Neurobiology, 15*(2), 231–238.

Price, G. R., & Ansari, D. (2011). Symbol processing in the left angular gyrus: Evidence from passive perception of digits. *NeuroImage.* Special Issue: Educational Neuroscience, *57*(3), 1205–1211.

Price, G. R., Holloway, I., Räsänen, P., Vesterinen, M., & Ansari, D. (2007). Impaired parietal magnitude processing in developmental dyscalculia. *Current Biology, 17*(24), R1042–R1043.

Price, G. R., Mazzocco, M. M. M., & Ansari, D. (2013). Why Mental Arithmetic Counts: Brain Activation during Single Digit Arithmetic Predicts High School Math Scores. *Journal of Neuroscience, 33*(1), 156–163.

Pugh, K. R., Mencl, W. E., Jenner, A. R., Katz, L., Frost, S. J., Lee, J. R., ... Shaywitz, B. A. (2000). Functional neuroimaging studies of reading and reading disability (developmental dyslexia). *Mental Retardation and Developmental Disabilities Research Reviews, 6*(3), 207–213.

Pugh, K. R., Mencl, W. E., Jenner, A. R., Katz, L., Frost, S. J., Lee, J. R., ... Shaywitz, B. A. (2001). Neurobiological studies of reading and reading disability. *Journal of Communication Disorders, 34*(6), 479–492.

Purcell, E. M., Torrey, H. C., & Pound, R. V. (1946). Resonance Absorption by Nuclear Magnetic Moments in a Solid. *Physical Review, 69*(1-2), 37–38.

Purpura, D. J., Logan, J. A. R., Hassinger-Das, B., & Napoli, A. R. (2017). Why do early mathematics skills predict later reading? The role of mathematical language. *Developmental Psychology, 53*(9), 1633–1642.

Qin, S., Cho, S., Chen, T., Rosenberg-Lee, M., Geary, D. C., & Menon, V. (2014). Hippocampal-neocortical functional reorganization underlies children's cognitive development. *Nature Neuroscience, 17*(9), 1263–1269.

R Core Team. (2016). R: A language and environment for statistical computing. Vienna, Austria: R Foundation for Statistical Computing. Retrieved from https://www.R-project.org/

Raghubar, K. P., Barnes, M. A., & Hecht, S. A. (2010). Working memory and mathematics: A review of developmental, individual difference, and cognitive approaches. *Learning and Individual Differences, 20*(2), 110–122.

Raichle, M. E. (2011). The Restless Brain. *Brain Connectivity, 1*(1), 3–12.

Ramus, F., Altarelli, I., Jednoróg, K., Zhao, J., & Scotto di Covella, L. (2018). Neuroanatomy of developmental dyslexia: Pitfalls and promise. *Neuroscience & Biobehavioral Reviews, 84*, 434–452.

Ramus, F., Rosen, S., Dakin, S. C., Day, B. L., Castellote, J. M., White, S., & Frith, U. (2003). Theories of developmental dyslexia: Insights from a multiple case study of dyslexic adults. *Brain, 126*(4), 841–865.

Ranpura, A., Isaacs, E., Edmonds, C., Rogers, M., Lanigan, J., Singhal, A., … Butterworth, B. (2013). Developmental trajectories of grey and white matter in dyscalculia. *Trends in Neuroscience and Education, 2*(2), 56–64.

Raschle, N. M., Chang, M., & Gaab, N. (2011). Structural brain alterations associated with dyslexia predate reading onset. *NeuroImage, 57*(3), 742–749.

Raybaud, C., Ahmad, T., Rastegar, N., Shroff, M., & Al Nassar, M. (2013). The premature brain: Developmental and lesional anatomy. *Neuroradiology, 55*(2), 23–40.

Reuter, M., & Fischl, B. (2011). Avoiding asymmetry-induced bias in longitudinal image processing. *NeuroImage, 57*(1), 19.

Reuter, M., Schmansky, N. J., Rosas, H. D., & Fischl, B. (2012). Within-subject template estimation for unbiased longitudinal image analysis. *NeuroImage, 61*(4), 1402–1418.

Richardson, U., Thomson, J. M., Scott, S. K., & Goswami, U. (2004). Auditory processing skills and phonological representation in dyslexic children. *Dyslexia, 10*(3), 215–233.

Richlan, F., Kronbichler, M., & Wimmer, H. (2009). Functional abnormalities in the dyslexic brain: A quantitative meta-analysis of neuroimaging studies. *Human Brain Mapping, 30*(10), 3299–3308.

Richlan, F., Kronbichler, M., & Wimmer, H. (2011). Meta-analyzing brain dysfunctions in dyslexic children and adults. *NeuroImage, 56*(3), 1735–1742.

Richlan, F., Kronbichler, M., & Wimmer, H. (2013). Structural abnormalities in the dyslexic brain: A meta-analysis of voxel-based morphometry studies. *Human Brain Mapping, 34*(11), 3055–3065.

Richman, D. P., Stewart, R. M., Hutchinson, J. W., & Caviness, V. S., Jr. (1975). Mechanical model of brain convolutional development. *Science, 189*, 18–21.

Rimrodt, S. L., Peterson, D. J., Denckla, M. B., Kaufmann, W. E., & Cutting, L. E. (2010). White matter microstructural differences linked to left perisylvian language network in children with dyslexia. *Cortex, 46*(6), 739–749.

Rivera, S. M., Reiss, A. L., Eckert, M. A., & Menon, V. (2005). Developmental changes in mental arithmetic: Evidence for increased functional specialization in the left inferior parietal cortex. *Cerebral Cortex, 15*(11), 1779–1790.

Ronan, L., Voets, N., Rua, C., Alexander-Bloch, A., Hough, M., Mackay, C., . . . Fletcher, P. C. (2014). Differential tangential expansion as a mechanism for cortical gyrification. *Cerebral Cortex*, 24(8), 2219–2228.

Rosen, S., & Manganari, E. (2001). Is there a relationship between speech and nonspeech auditory processing in children with dyslexia? *Journal of Speech Language and Hearing Research*, 44(4), 720–736.

Rosenberg-Lee, M., Chang, T. T., Young, C. B., Wu, S., & Menon, V. (2011). Functional dissociations between four basic arithmetic operations in the human posterior parietal cortex: A cytoarchitectonic mapping study. *Neuropsychologia*, 49(9), 2592–2608.

Rotzer, S., Kucian, K., Martin, E., von Aster, M., Klaver, P., & Loenneker, T. (2008). Optimized voxel-based morphometry in children with developmental dyscalculia. *NeuroImage*, 39(1), 417–422.

Rotzer, S., Loenneker, T., Kucian, K., Martin, E., Klaver, P., & von Aster, M. (2009). Dysfunctional neural network of spatial working memory contributes to developmental dyscalculia. *Neuropsychologia*, 47(13), 2859–2865.

Salmelin, R. E., Service, E., Kiesilä, P., Uutela, K., & Salonen, O. (1996). Impaired visual word processing in dyslexia revealed with magnetoencephalography: Visual word recognition. *Annals of Neurology*, 40(2), 157–162.

Sammons, L. (2011). *Building mathematical comprehension: Using literacy strategies to make meaning* (D. Herweck Rice, S. Johnson, & H. Wolfe, Eds.). Shell Education.

Sammons, P., Elliot, K., Sylva, K., Melhuish, E., Siraj-Blatchford, I., & Taggart, B. (2004). The impact of pre-school on young children's cognitive attainments at entry to reception. *British Educational Research Journal*, 30(5), 691–712.

Savage, R. S., Frederickson, N., Goodwin, R., Patni, U., Smith, N., & Tuersley, L. (2005). Relationships among rapid digit naming, phonological processing, motor automaticity, and speech perception in poor, average, and good readers and spellers. *Journal of Learning Disabilities*, 38(1), 12–28.

Saygin, Z. M., Norton, E. S., Osher, D. E., Beach, S. D., Cyr, A. B., Ozernov-Palchik, O., . . . Gabrieli, J. D. E. (2013). Tracking the roots of reading ability: White matter volume and integrity correlate with phonological awareness in prereading and early-reading kindergarten children. *Journal of Neuroscience*, 33(33), 13251–13258.

Schaadt, G., Männel, C., van der Meer, E., Pannekamp, A., Oberecker, R., & Friederici, A. D. (2015). Present and past: Can writing abilities in school children be associated with their auditory discrimination capacities in infancy? *Research in Developmental Disabilities*, 47, 318–333.

Schaer, M., Glaser, B., Cuadra, M. B., Debbane, M., Thiran, J.-P., & Eliez, S. (2009). Congenital heart disease affects local gyrification in 22q11.2 deletion syndrome. *Developmental Medicine & Child Neurology*, 51(9), 746–753.

Schlaggar, B. L., & McCandliss, B. D. (2007). Development of Neural Systems for Reading. *Annual Review of Neuroscience*, 30(1), 475–503.

Schöpf, V., Kasprian, G., Brugger, P. C., & Prayer, D. (2012). Watching the fetal brain at 'rest'. *International Journal of Developmental Neuroscience*, 30(1), 11–17.

Schreiber, J., Riffert, T., Anwander, A., & Knösche, T. R. (2014). Plausibility Tracking: A method to evaluate anatomical connectivity and microstructural properties along fiber pathways. *NeuroImage, 90*, 163–178.

Schulte-Körne, G. (2010). The prevention, diagnosis, and treatment of dyslexia. *Deutsches Ärzteblatt International, 107*(41), 718–727.

Schwanenflugel, P. J., Meisinger, E. B., Wisenbaker, J. M., Kuhn, M. R., Strauss, G. P., & Morris, R. D. (2006). Becoming a fluent and automatic reader in the early elementary school years. *Reading Research Quarterly, 41*(4), 496–522.

Scientific and Statistical Computing Core. (2017). Analysis of Functional Neuroimages software. Bethesda, MD, US: National Institute of Mental Health.

Ségonne, F., Dale, A. M., Busa, E., Glessner, M., Salat, D., Hahn, H. K., & Fischl, B. (2004). A hybrid approach to the skull stripping problem in MRI. *NeuroImage, 22*(3), 1060–1075.

Seidenberg, M. S., & McClelland, J. L. (1989). A distributed, developmental model of word recognition and naming. *Psychological Review, 96*(4), 523.

Shaw, P., Eckstrand, K., Sharp, W., Blumenthal, J., Lerch, J. P., Greenstein, D., . . . Rapoport, J. L. (2007). Attention-deficit/hyperactivity disorder is characterized by a delay in cortical maturation. *Proceedings of the National Academy of Sciences of the United States of America, 104*(49), 19649–19654.

Shaw, P., Greenstein, D., Lerch, J. P., Clasen, L., Lenroot, R. K., Gogtay, N., . . . Giedd, J. N. (2006). Intellectual ability and cortical development in children and adolescents. *Nature, 440*(7084), 676–679.

Shaw, P., Kabani, N. J., Lerch, J. P., Eckstrand, K., Lenroot, R. K., Gogtay, N., . . . Wise, S. P. (2008). Neurodevelopmental trajectories of the human cerebral cortex. *Journal of Neuroscience, 28*(14), 3586–3594.

Shaywitz, B. A., Shaywitz, S. E., Pugh, K. R., Mencl, W. E., Fulbright, R. K., Skudlarski, P., . . . Gore, J. C. (2002). Disruption of posterior brain systems for reading in children with developmental dyslexia. *Biological Psychiatry, 52*(2), 101–110.

Shaywitz, S. E. (1998). Dyslexia. *New England Journal of Medicine, 338*(5), 307–312.

Shaywitz, S. E., Shaywitz, B. A., Fulbright, R. K., Skudlarski, P., Mencl, W. E., Constable, R. T., . . . Gore, J. C. (2003). Neural systems for compensation and persistence: Young adult outcome of childhood reading disability. *Biological Psychiatry, 54*(1), 25–33.

Shaywitz, S. E., Shaywitz, B. A., Pugh, K. R., Fulbright, R. K., Constable, R. T., Mencl, W. E., . . . Gore, J. C. (1998). Functional disruption in the organization of the brain for reading in dyslexia. *Proceedings of the National Academy of Sciences of the United States of America, 95*(5), 2636–2641.

Shum, J., Hermes, D., Foster, B. L., Dastjerdi, M., Rangarajan, V., Winawer, J., . . . Parvizi, J. (2013). A Brain Area for Visual Numerals. *Journal of Neuroscience, 33*(16), 6709–6715.

Siegel, S. (1956). *Nonparametric statistics for the behavioral sciences.* Nonparametric statistics for the behavioral sciences. New York, NY, US: McGraw-Hill.

Siegler, R. S., & Shipley, C. (1995). Variation, selection, and cognitive change. In T. Simon & G. Halford (Eds.), *Developing cognitive competence: New approaches to process modeling* (pp. 31–76). Hillsdale, NJ, US: Lawrence Erlbaum Associates, Inc.

Silani, G., Frith, U., Démonet, J.-F., Fazio, F., Perani, D., Price, C. J., ... Paulesu, E. (2005). Brain abnormalities underlying altered activation in dyslexia: A voxel based morphometry study. *Brain, 128*(10), 2453–2461.

Simon, O., Mangin, J.-F., Cohen, L., Le Bihan, D., & Dehaene, S. (2002). Topographical layout of hand, eye, calculation, and language-related areas in the human parietal lobe. *Neuron, 33*(3), 475–487.

Skeide, M. A., Brauer, J., & Friederici, A. D. (2016). Brain functional and structural predictors of language performance. *Cerebral Cortex, 26*(5), 2127–2139.

Skeide, M. A., Evans, T. M., Mei, E. Z., Abrams, D. A., & Menon, V. (2018). Neural signatures of co-occurring reading and mathematical difficulties. *Developmental Science, 21*(6), e12680.

Skeide, M. A., Kirsten, H., Kraft, I., Schaadt, G., Müller, B., Neef, N. E., ... Friederici, A. D. (2015). Genetic dyslexia risk variant is related to neural connectivity patterns underlying phonological awareness in children. *NeuroImage, 118*, 414–421.

Skeide, M. A., Kumar, U., Mishra, R. K., Tripathi, V. N., Guleria, A., Singh, J. P., ... Huettig, F. (2017). Learning to read alters cortico-subcortical cross-talk in the visual system of illiterates. *Science Advances, 3*(5), e1602612.

Skoglund, T. S., Pascher, R., & Berthold, C.-H. (1996). Heterogeneity in the columnar number of neurons in different neocortical areas in the rat. *Neuroscience Letters, 208*(2), 97–100.

Slaughter, V., Kamppi, D., & Paynter, J. (2006). Toddler subtraction with large sets: Further evidence for an analog-magnitude representation of number. *Developmental Science, 9*(1), 33–39.

Smith, E. E., & Jonides, J. (1998). Neuroimaging analyses of human working memory. *Proceedings of the National Academy of Sciences of the United States of America, 95*(20), 12061–12068.

Smith, S. M., Jenkinson, M., Johansen-Berg, H., Rueckert, D., Nichols, T. E., Mackay, C. E., ... Behrens, T. E. (2006). Tract-based spatial statistics: Voxelwise analysis of multi-subject diffusion data. *NeuroImage, 31*(4), 1487–1505.

Smith, S. M., Jenkinson, M., Woolrich, M. W., Beckmann, C. F., Behrens, T. E. J., Johansen-Berg, H., ... Matthews, P. M. (2004). Advances in functional and structural MR image analysis and implementation as FSL. *NeuroImage, 23*, S208–S219.

Snowling, M. J. (1998). Dyslexia as a phonological deficit: Evidence and implications. *Child Psychology and Psychiatry Review, 3*(1), 4–11.

Snowling, M. J., Muter, V., & Carroll, J. (2007). Children at family risk of dyslexia: A follow-up in early adolescence. *Journal of Child Psychology and Psychiatry, 48*(6), 609–618.

Soares, J. M., Marques, P., Alves, V., & Sousa, N. (2013). A hitchhiker's guide to diffusion tensor imaging. *Frontiers in Neuroscience, 7*, 31.

Song, M., Zhou, Y., Li, J., Liu, Y., Tian, L., Yu, C., & Jiang, T. (2008). Brain spontaneous functional connectivity and intelligence. *NeuroImage, 41*(3), 1168–1176.

Sowell, E., Thompson, P. M., Leonard, C. M., Welcome, S. E., Kan, E., & Toga, A. W. (2004). Longitudinal mapping of cortical thickness and brain growth in normal children. *Journal of Neuroscience, 24*(38), 8223–8231.

Spinelli, D., De Luca, M., Judica, A., & Zoccolotti, P. (2002). Crowding effects on word identification in developmental dyslexia. *Cortex, 38*(2), 179–200.

SPM12. (2016). Wellcome Centre for Human Neuroimaging. Retrieved from https://www.fil.ion.ucl.ac.uk/spm/software/spm12

Stauder, A. (2010). The earliest egyptian writing. In C. Woods, G. Emberling, & E. Teeter (Eds.), *Visible language: Inventions of writing in the ancient Middle East and beyond* (no. 32, pp. 137–148). Oriental Institute Museum publications. Chicago, Ill: Oriental Institute of the University of Chicago.

Stein, J. F. (2001). The magnocellular theory of developmental dyslexia. *Dyslexia, 7*(1), 12–36.

Stein, J. F. (2018). The current status of the magnocellular theory of developmental dyslexia. *Neuropsychologia.*

Stein, J. F., & Talcott, J. B. (1999). Impaired neuronal timing in developmental dyslexia—the magnocellular hypothesis. *Dyslexia, 5*(2), 59–77.

Stein, J. F., & Walsh, V. (1997). To see but not to read; the magnocellular theory of dyslexia. *Trends in Neurosciences, 20*(4), 147–152.

Stejskal, E. O., & Tanner, J. E. (1965). Spin Diffusion Measurements: Spin Echoes in the Presence of a Time-Dependent Field Gradient. *The Journal of Chemical Physics, 42*(1), 288–292.

Stevens, M. C., Pearlson, G. D., & Calhoun, V. D. (2009). Changes in the interaction of resting-state neural networks from adolescence to adulthood. *Human Brain Mapping, 30*(8), 2356–2366.

Stiles, J., & Jernigan, T. L. (2010). The basics of brain developmet. *Neuropsychology Review, 20*(4), 327–348.

Stock, C., Marx, H., & Schneider, W. (2003). *BAKO 1–4: Basiskompetenzen für Lese-Rechtschreibleistungen.* Göttingen: Hogrefe.

Stock, C., & Schneider, W. (2008). *DERET 1–2+: Deutscher Rechtschreibtest für das erste und zweite Schuljahr.* Göttingen: Hogrefe.

Stoodley, C. J., Ray, N. J., Jack, A., & Stein, J. F. (2008). Implicit learning in control, dyslexic, and garden-variety poor readers. *Annals of the New York Academy of Sciences, 1145*(1), 173–183.

Supekar, K., Swigart, A. G., Tenison, C., Jolles, D. D., Rosenberg-Lee, M., Fuchs, L., & Menon, V. (2013). Neural predictors of individual differences in response to math tutoring in primary-grade school children. *Proceedings of the National Academy of Sciences of the United States of America, 110*(20), 8230–8235.

Tallal, P. (1980). Auditory temporal perception, phonics, and reading disabilities in children. *Brain and Language, 9*(2), 182–198.

Tallinen, T., Chung, J. Y., Rousseau, F., Girard, N., Lefèvre, J., & Mahadevan, L. (2016). On the growth and form of cortical convolutions. *Nature Physics, 12*(6), 588–593.

Tardif, C. L., Schäfer, A., Trampel, R., Villringer, A., Turner, R., & Bazin, P.-L. (2016). Open Science CBS Neuroimaging Repository: Sharing ultra-high-field MR images of the brain. *NeuroImage*. Sharing the wealth: Brain Imaging Repositories in 2015, *124*, 1143–1148.

Tau, G. Z., & Peterson, B. S. (2010). Normal development of brain circuits. *Neuropsychopharmacology*, *35*(1), 147–168.

The MathWorks, Inc. (2017). MATLAB. Natick, MA, USA: The Mathworks, Inc.

Thomason, M. E., Dassanayake, M. T., Shen, S., Katkuri, Y., Alexis, M., Anderson, A. L., . . . Romero, R. (2013). Cross-hemispheric functional connectivity in the human fetal brain. *Science Translational Medicine*, *5*(173), 173ra24.

Thompson, L. A., Detterman, D. K., & Plomin, R. (1991). Associations between cognitive abilities and scholastic achievement: Genetic overlap but environmental differences. *Psychological Science*, *2*(3), 158–165.

Thornburgh, C. L., Narayana, S., Rezaie, R., Bydlinski, B. N., Tylavsky, F. A., Papanicolaou, A. C., . . . Völgyi, E. (2017). Concordance of the resting state networks in typically developing, 6-to 7-year-old children and healthy adults. *Frontiers in Human Neuroscience*, *11*, 199.

Tian, L., Ren, J., & Zang, Y.-F. (2012). Regional homogeneity of resting state fMRI signals predicts stop signal task performance. *NeuroImage*, *60*(1), 539–544.

Tisserand, D. J., van Boxtel, M. P. J., Pruessner, J. C., Hofman, P., Evans, A. C., & Jolles, J. (2004). A voxel-based morphometric study to determine individual differences in gray matter density associated with age and cognitive change over time. *Cerebral Cortex*, *14*(9), 966–973.

Tosun, D., Rettmann, M. E., Han, X., Tao, X., Xu, C., Resnick, S. M., . . . Prince, J. L. (2004). Cortical surface segmentation and mapping. *NeuroImage*, *23*, S108–S118.

Tournier, J.-D., Mori, S., & Leemans, A. (2011). Diffusion tensor imaging and beyond. *Magnetic Resonance in Medicine*, *65*(6), 1532–1556.

Van Essen, D. C. (1997). A tension-based theory of morphogenesis and compact wiring in the central nervous system. *Nature*, *385*(6614), 313–318.

van Atteveldt, N., Formisano, E., Goebel, R., & Blomert, L. (2004). Integration of letters and speech sounds in the human brain. *Neuron*, *43*(2), 271–282.

van Oers, C. A. M. M., Goldberg, N., Fiorin, G., van den Heuvel, M. P., Kappelle, L. J., & Wijnen, F. N. K. (2018). No evidence for cerebellar abnormality in adults with developmental dyslexia. *Experimental Brain Research*, *236*(11), 2991–3001.

van Zuijen, T. L., Plakas, A., Maassen, B. A. M., Maurits, N. M., & van der Leij, A. (2013). Infant ERPs separate children at risk of dyslexia who become good readers from those who become poor readers. *Developmental Science*, *16*(4), 554–563.

Vandermosten, M., Boets, B., Poelmans, H., Sunaert, S., Wouters, J., & Ghesquière, P. (2012). A tractography study in dyslexia: Neuroanatomic correlates of orthographic, phonological and speech processing. *Brain*, *135*(3), 935–948.

Vandermosten, M., Vanderauwera, J., Theys, C., De Vos, A., Vanvooren, S., Sunaert, S., . . . Ghesquière, P. (2015). A DTI tractography study in pre-readers at risk for dyslexia. *Developmental Cognitive Neuroscience*, *14*, 8–15.

Vellutino, F. R., Fletcher, J. M., Snowling, M. J., & Scanlon, D. M. (2004). Specific reading disability (dyslexia): What have we learned in the past four decades? *Journal of Child Psychology and Psychiatry*, *45*(1), 2–40.

Venkatraman, V., Ansari, D., & Chee, M. W. L. (2005). Neural correlates of symbolic and non-symbolic arithmetic. *Neuropsychologia, 43*(5), 744–753.

Vicari, S., Marotta, L., Menghini, D., Molinari, M., & Petrosini, L. (2003). Implicit learning deficit in children with developmental dyslexia. *Neuropsychologia, 41*(1), 108–114.

Visser, M., Jefferies, E., & Lambon Ralph, M. A. (2010). Semantic processing in the anterior temporal lobes: A meta-analysis of the functional neuroimaging literature. *Journal of Cognitive Neuroscience, 22*(6), 1083–1094.

von Aster, M., Schweiter, M., & Weinhold Zulauf, M. (2007). Rechenstörungen bei Kindern. *Zeitschrift für Entwicklungspsychologie und Pädagogische Psychologie, 39*(2), 85–96.

von Economo, C. F., & Koskinas, G. N. (1925). *Die Cytoarchitektonik der Hirnrinde des erwachsenen Menschen.* Berlin: Julius Springer.

Wadsworth, S. J., DeFries, J. C., Fulker, D. W., & Plomin, R. (1995). Cognitive ability and academic achievement in the Colorado Adoption Project: A multivariate genetic analysis of parent-offspring and sibling data. *Behavior Genetics, 25*(1), 1–15.

Wadsworth, S. J., Olson, R. K., & DeFries, J. C. (2010). Differential genetic etiology of reading difficulties as a function of IQ: An update. *Behavior genetics, 40*(6), 751–758.

Wagstyl, K., & Lerch, J. P. (2018). Cortical thickness. In G. Spalletta, F. Piras, & T. Gili (Eds.), *Brain morphometry* (pp. 35–49). New York, NY, US: Humana Press.

Wagstyl, K., Ronan, L., Goodyer, I. M., & Fletcher, P. C. (2015). Cortical thickness gradients in structural hierarchies. *NeuroImage, 111*, 241–250.

Walhovd, K. B., Fjell, A. M., Giedd, J. N., Dale, A. M., & Brown, T. T. (2016). Through thick and thin: A need to reconcile contradictory results on trajectories in human cortical development. *Cerebral Cortex, 27*(2), 1472–1481.

Wechsler, D., Petermann, F., & Lipsius, M. (2009). *WPPSI-III: Wechsler preschool and primary scale of intelligence. German Version.* Frankfurt am Main: Pearson Assessment.

Westbrook, C., & Talbot, J. (2019). *MRI in Practice.* John Wiley & Sons Ltd.

White, S., Frith, U., Milne, E., Rosen, S., Swettenham, J., & Ramus, F. (2006). A double dissociation between sensorimotor impairments and reading disability: A comparison of autistic and dyslexic children. *Cognitive Neuropsychology, 23*(5), 748–761.

White, T., Su, S., Schmidt, M., Kao, C.-Y., & Sapiro, G. (2010). The development of gyrification in childhood and adolescence. *Brain and Cognition, 72*(1), 36–45.

Williams, M. J., Stuart, G. W., Castles, A., & McAnally, K. I. (2003). Contrast sensitivity in subgroups of developmental dyslexia. *Vision Research, 43*(4), 467–477.

Woods, C. (2010). The earliest mesopotamian writing. In C. Woods, G. Emberling, & E. Teeter (Eds.), *Visible language: Inventions of writing in the ancient Middle East and beyond* (no. 32, pp. 33–84). Oriental Institute Museum publications. Chicago, Ill: Oriental Institute of the University of Chicago.

World Health Organization. (2018). *ICD-11 International classification of diseases for mortality and morbidity statistics. Eleventh revision.*

World Medical Association. (2013). World Medical Association declaration of Helsinki: Ethical principles for medical research involving human subjects, 2191–2194.

Xu, F., & Spelke, E. S. (2000). Large number discrimination in 6-month-old infants. *Cognition, 74*(1), B1–B11.

Xu, G., Knutsen, A. K., Dikranian, K., Kroenke, C. D., Bayly, P. V., & Taber, L. A. (2010). Axons pull on the brain, but tension does not drive cortical folding. *Journal of Biomechanical Engineering, 132*(7), 071013.

Yan, C.-G., & Zang, Y.-F. (2010). DPARSF: A MATLAB toolbox for "pipeline" data analysis of resting-state fMRI. *Frontiers in Systems Neuroscience, 4*, 13.

Yeatman, J. D., Dougherty, R. F., Ben-Shachar, M., & Wandell, B. A. (2012). Development of white matter and reading skills. *Proceedings of the National Academy of Sciences of the United States of America, 109*(44), E3045–E3053.

Yeniad, N., Malda, M., Mesman, J., van Ijzendoorn, M. H., & Pieper, S. (2013). Shifting ability predicts math and reading performance in children: A meta-analytical study. *Learning and Individual Differences, 23*, 1–9.

Yeo, D. J., Wilkey, E. D., & Price, G. R. (2017). The search for the number form area: A functional neuroimaging meta-analysis. *Neuroscience & Biobehavioral Reviews, 78*, 145–160.

Yin, S., Zhu, X., Li, R., Niu, Y., Wang, B., Zheng, Z., . . . Li, J. (2014). Intervention-induced enhancement in intrinsic brain activity in healthy older adults. *Scientific Reports, 4*, 7309.

Yoon, U., Fonov, V. S., Perusse, D., Evans, A. C., & Brain Development Cooperative Group. (2009). The effect of template choice on morphometric analysis of pediatric brain data. *NeuroImage, 45*(3), 769–777.

Yotter, R. A., Dahnke, R., Thompson, P. M., & Gaser, C. (2011). Topological correction of brain surface meshes using spherical harmonics. *Human Brain Mapping, 32*(7), 1109–1124.

Yotter, R. A., Nenadic, I., Ziegler, G., Thompson, P. M., & Gaser, C. (2011). Local cortical surface complexity maps from spherical harmonic reconstructions. *NeuroImage, 56*(3), 961–973.

Yotter, R. A., Thompson, P. M., & Gaser, C. (2011). Algorithms to improve the reparameterization of spherical mappings of brain surface meshes. *Journal of Neuroimaging, 21*(2), e134–e147.

Zang, Y.-F., Jiang, T., Lu, Y., He, Y., & Tian, L. (2004). Regional homogeneity approach to fMRI data analysis. *NeuroImage, 22*(1), 394–400.

Zatorre, R. J., Fields, R. D., & Johansen-Berg, H. (2012). Plasticity in gray and white: Neuroimaging changes in brain structure during learning. *Nature Neuroscience, 15*(4), 528–536.

Zhang, M., Li, J., Chen, C., Xue, G., Lu, Z., Mei, L., . . . Dong, Q. (2014). Resting-state functional connectivity and reading abilities in first and second languages. *NeuroImage, 84*, 546–553.

Zhang, T., Razavi, M. J., Li, X., Chen, H., Liu, T., & Wang, X. (2016). Mechanism of consistent gyrus formation: An experimental and computational study. *Scientific Reports, 6*(1), 6:37272.

Zhang, Y., Brady, M., & Smith, S. M. (2001). Segmentation of brain MR images through a hidden Markov random field model and the expectation-maximization algorithm. *IEEE Transactions on Medical Imaging*, *20*(1), 45–57.

Ziegler, J. C., Bertrand, D., Tóth, D., Csépe, V., Reis, A., Faísca, L., ... Blomert, L. (2010). Orthographic depth and its impact on universal predictors of reading: A cross-language investigation. *Psychological Science*, *21*(4), 551–559.

Zorzi, M., Houghton, G., & Butterworth, B. (1998). Two routes or one in reading aloud? A connectionist dual-process model. *Journal of Experimental Psychology: Human Perception and Performance*, *24*(4), 1131–1161.

Zou, Q.-H., Zhu, C.-Z., Yang, Y., Zuo, X.-N., Long, X.-Y., Cao, Q.-J., ... Zang, Y.-F. (2008). An improved approach to detection of amplitude of low-frequency fluctuation (ALFF) for resting-state fMRI: Fractional ALFF. *Journal of Neuroscience Methods*, *172*(1), 137–141.

Zuo, X.-N., Di Martino, A., Kelly, C., Shehzad, Z. E., Gee, D. G., Klein, D. F., ... Milham, M. P. (2010). The oscillating brain: Complex and reliable. *NeuroImage*, *49*(2), 1432–1445.

Zuo, X.-N., Xu, T., Jiang, L., Yang, Z., Cao, X.-Y., He, Y., ... Milham, M. P. (2013). Toward reliable characterization of functional homogeneity in the human brain: Preprocessing, scan duration, imaging resolution and computational space. *NeuroImage*, *65*, 374–386.

CURRICULUM VITAE

PERSONAL DETAILS

Name	Ulrike Kuhl
Date of birth	19. February 1990
Place of birth	Löningen

EDUCATION

since 10/2014	PhD student
	Department of Neuropsychology
	Max Planck Institute for Human
	Cognitive and Brain Sciences
	Leipzig, Germany
07/2016 - 08/2016	Medical Imaging Summer School
	Favignana, Italy
10/2012 - 09/2014	M.Sc. Cognitive Science
	Institute of Cognitive Science
	University of Osnabrück
	Osnabrück, Germany
09/2011 - 12/2011	Semester abroad
	University College Dublin
	Dublin, Ireland
10/2009 - 09/2012	B.Sc. Cognitive Science
	Institute of Cognitive Science
	University of Osnabrück
	Osnabrück, Germany

06/2009   Abitur (A-levels)

                            Artland Gymnasium Quakenbrück

                            Quakenbrück, Germany

PROFESSIONAL EXPERIENCE

09/2013 - 09/2014   Research assistant

                            Department of Psycho- and

                            Neurolinguistics

                            Institute of Cognitive Science

                            University of Osnabrück

                            Osnabrück Germany

09/2013 - 09/2014   Teaching assistant

                            Department of Neurobiopsychology

                            Institute of Cognitive Science

                            University of Osnabrück

                            Osnabrück Germany

04/2012 - 09/2014   Teaching assistant

                            Department of Philosophy of

                            Mind and Cognition

                            Institute of Cognitive Science

                            University of Osnabrück

                            Osnabrück Germany

PUBLICATIONS & TALKS

INTERNATIONAL JOURNAL ARTICLES

Jeon, H.-A., **Kuhl, U.**, & Friederici, A.D. *Mathematical expertise modulates the architecture of dorsal and cortico-thalamic white matter tracts.* Scientific reports, 9(1), 6825.

Kuhl, U., Friederici, A.D., the LEGASCREEN consortium & Skeide, M.A. *Early cortical surface plasticity relates to basic mathematical learning.* Manuscript submitted for publication.

Kuhl, U., Neef, N.E., Kraft, I., Schaadt, G., Dörr, L., Brauer, J., Czepezauer, I., Müller, B., Wilcke, A., Kirsten, H., Emmrich, F., Boltze, J., Friederici, A.D., & Skeide, M.A. *Neurobiological origins of developmental dyslexia.* Manuscript submitted for publication.

TALKS

Kuhl, U. (2019, September). *Neurobiological correlates of individual differences in mathematical development.* Talk presented at the Mittweida Workshop on Computational Intelligence, Mittweida, Germany.

Kuhl, U. (2019, August). The neurobiological predisposition for developing dyslexia. In M.A. Skeide (Chair), *Neurocognitive origins of learning disorders.* Symposium conducted at the meeting of the European Association for Research on Learning and Instruction (EARLI), Aachen, Germany.

Kuhl, U. (2018, November). *Detecting cortical facets of developmental disorders using multivariate random forest classification: the case of dyslexia.* Talk presented at the Research Institute for Cognition and Robotics, University of Bielefeld, Bielefeld, Germany.

Kuhl, U. (2017, April). *Disentangling sensory deficit theories of dyslexia: insights from diffusion and structural MRI.* Talk presented at the Max Planck Institute for Human Cognitive and Brain Sciences, Leipzig, Germany.

POSTER PRESENTATIONS

Kuhl, U., Friederici, A.D., & Skeide, M.A. (2017, November). *The Dyslexic Brain Before and After Literacy: Unifying Structural Signs.* Poster presented at the 9th annual meeting of Society for the Neurobiology of Language, Baltimore, MD, USA.

Kuhl, U., Friederici, A.D., & Skeide, M.A. (2017, November). *Detecting Cortical Facets of Developmental Disorders using Multivariate Random Forest Classification: The Case of Dyslexia.* Poster presented at the 47th annual meeting of the Society for Neuroscience, Washington DC, USA.

Kuhl, U., Friederici, A.D., & Skeide, M.A. (2017, September). *The Dyslexic Brain Before and After Literacy: Unifying Structural Signs.* Poster session presented at the Visions in Science, Berlin, Germany.

Kuhl, U., Friederici, A.D., & Skeide, M.A. (2017, September). *The Dyslexic Brain Before and After Literacy: Unifying Structural Signs.* Poster session presented at the 23rd Conference on Architectures and Mechanisms of Language Processing, Lancaster, UK.

Kuhl, U., Friederici, A.D., & Jeon, H.–A. (2017, June). *Being an Expert Reflected by Structural Connectivity: A Tractography Study on Mathematical Expertise.* Poster session presented at the 23rd annual meeting of the Organization for Human Brain Mapping, Vancouver, BC, Canada.

SUMMARY OF DISSERTATION

Reliable early literacy and numeracy abilities provide the foundation of more complex, high level skills (Geary, 2011) and successful academic achievement (Duncan et al., 2007). However, not all individuals acquire abilities such as reading, writing and arithmetic with the same ease (M. Brown et al., 2003; Cockcroft, 1982). Importantly, the neural origins of behavioural differences in such complex cognitive skills still represent a matter of debate.

Research into specific neural correlates of literacy and numeracy has proven challenging. First, longitudinal experimental designs starting before school are necessary to identify neurobiological profiles and developmental changes directly related to behavioural variation (Goswami, 2015; Ramus et al., 2018). Thus far, however, longitudinal evidence is sparse. Second, the considerable covariation between literacy or numeracy skills (Durand et al., 2005; Hart et al., 2009) has to be taken into account when studying specific correlates of distinct abilities. Third, a more integrated approach combining various anatomical and functional dimensions may be needed to provide a comprehensive under-standing of the emergence of complex cognitive abilities and their developmental trajectories.

The aim of the present dissertation was to shed light on neu-ral development supporting early literacy and numeracy. To this end, we investigated the brain basis of these complex cognitive abilities using structural and resting-state functional magnetic resonance imaging. Specifically, this thesis focuses on two cen-tral questions: What are the neural correlates of *(a)* deficient lit-eracy acquisition and *(b)* individual differences in mathematical development? Both questions were investigated using longitu-dinal data acquired from children undergoing a comprehensive series of psychometric testing and neuroimaging from kinder-garten until the end of second grade in school, i. e. at 5 and 8 years of age. Following participants over this period of time re-vealed specific neurobiological profiles related to individual be-havioural variation. What is more, the presented analyses quan-tified diverse neuroanatomical and -functional measures, while controlling for pertinent covariates including sociodemographic status, intellectual abilities and individual performance in liter-acy and numeracy.

The first empirical study presented in this thesis aimed to sys-tematically test whether existing neurobiological theories of developmental dyslexia reflect potential neural causes rather than consequences of impoverished literacy experience. In fact, various accounts suggesting neurobiological origins of specific literacy impairments exist. These range from deficits in auditory (Díaz et al., 2012; Hornickel & Kraus, 2013) or visual (Eden et al., 1996; Livingstone et al., 1991) pathways, over more general magnocellular defects (Stein, 2001; Stein & Walsh, 1997) and theories of cerebellar deficits (Nicolson et al., 2001), to higher-order processing impairments within the phonological speech processing system (Boets et al., 2013; S. E. Shaywitz et al., 1998). However, formulated claims are primarily based on data of adult or school-aged participants. Therefore, observed differences between cases and controls might be driven by a disparate amount and quality of literacy experience (Goswami, 2015; Ramus et al., 2018). To circumvent this issue, resting-state functional magnetic resonance imaging, T_1- and diffusion-weighted imaging data were acquired before and after literacy instruction in school. Based on standardised reading and writing measures acquired at school age, 16 children were classified as dyslexic and 16 as typically developing controls. Structural and functional measures characterizing complex cortical and subcortical networks that were previously linked to the aetiology of developmental dyslexia were subsequently compared.

The results show converging evidence for cortical malformation and reduced functional coherence within the speech processing system in individuals that develop literacy impairments. Specifically, future dyslexics' left primary auditory cortex exhibited higher degrees of cortical folding complexity both before and after first formal literacy instruction. Additionally, transient differences between dyslexic and typically developing children were detected when comparing structural and functional connectivity of left perisylvian regions. These effects included increased connectivity strength of the arcuate fasciculus connecting the planum temporale and Brodmann area 6 and reduced functional connectivity between the left primary auditory cortex and the planum temporale. Finally, prospective classification models based on the neural indices identified in the analysis proved above-chance discriminatory power, both alone or in combination with behavioural predictors. These findings extend the currently sparse evidence of neuroanatomical anomalies within the speech processing system of preliterate dyslexic children (Clark et al., 2014). Thereby, the current data supports the phonological deficit theory, suggesting that poor phonological skills impede the formation of reliable associations between letters and their corresponding sounds (Snowling, 1998). A speculative neurodevelopmental scenario I suggest based on the cur-

rent results may be that atypical gyrification of the primary auditory cortex and disrupted functional coherence between regions
within Heschl's gyrus mark aberrant neural migration. Consequently, the observed differences of the arcuate fasciculus might
present a secondary result arising from compensatory articulatory recoding strategies supported by the ventral premotor cortex (Pugh et al., 2000; Richlan et al., 2011; S. E. Shaywitz et al.,
1998). Still, subsequent studies based on larger populations of
dyslexic children are required to validate the current findings
and to evaluate their generalizability to other, non-alphabetic or
less transparent orthographies.

   In the second empirical study, we investigated how cortical
surface plasticity from the last year of kindergarten until the second grade in school systematically covaries with performance in
arithmetic and visuospatial magnitude processing tasks at eight
years of age. To this end, data from a sample of 28 children without any developmental learning disorders were assessed longitudinally. Previous research emphasised the role of structural and
functional plasticity of core magnitude processing areas in the
right posterior parietal cortex (Cantlon et al., 2006; Menon, 2010;
Rivera et al., 2005) for typical numeracy development. Additionally, more immature processing has been linked to a greater reliance on regions associated with auxiliary functions including

working memory and attention (i. e. prefrontal cortex regions; Rivera et al., 2005). With age and experience, the contribution of these processes to numerical cognition diminishes, while the functional specialisation of the left posterior parietal cortex increases (Rivera et al., 2005). Additionally, involvement of the medial temporal lobe during mathematical processing is thought to reflect the initial development and subsequent consolidation of memory-based retrieval strategies for mathematical problem solving (Qin et al., 2014).

The results of the second study reveal links between early arithmetic and visuospatial magnitude processing, two fundamental aspects of basic numeracy skills, and cortical surface reorganisation within right-hemispheric regions. Specifically, arithmetic abilities significantly correlated with plasticity of cortical folding complexity of the right intraparietal sulcus and cortical thickness of the anterior temporal pole. At the same time, visuospatial magnitude processing skills were significantly associated with changes in cortical thickness within the right superior parietal lobe and the precentral gyrus, as well as with cortical folding complexity plasticity of the middle frontal gyrus. By highlighting differential contributions of right parietal divisions for distinct subcomponents of numeracy skill, the current results lend support from a very young age group to a characterisation of the intraparietal sulcus as a domain specific region housing core magnitude representations, and the superior parietal lobe as an area involved in visuospatial attention orienting (Dehaene et al., 2003). Further, the observed effects in regions associated with working memory are in line with studies demonstrating that working memory explains a substantial proportion of the variance of individual performance in mathematical tasks (Raghubar et al., 2010). Based on the fact that all significant effects reported in the second study were confined to the right hemisphere, I suggest that right-hemispheric processes promote initial numeracy development, while involvement of the left hemisphere increases with age and experience. This view is in line with findings from the literature in school-aged children (Rivera et al., 2005), but has to be further corroborated in future work.

Taken together, the current dissertation sheds light onto the developmental trajectories underlying literacy deficits and numeracy development, making a substantial step towards a more comprehensive understanding of how complex cognitive skills emerge and how specific disruptions may impair learning. The presented evidence suggests that acquisition and maturation of these abilities reshapes the circuitries for domain-specific as well as domain-general auxiliary functions (i. e. magnitude, visuospatial and working memory processing in numeracy), and that disruptions in regions supporting very specific aspects of complex processes may bear severe consequences for learning success (i. e. disruptions of the phonological system impeding literacy development).

ZUSAMMENFASSUNG DER DISSERTATION

Der erfolgreiche Erwerb von Lese-, Schreib- und Rechenkompetenzen bildet die Grundlage für komplexere Fähigkeiten (Geary,
2011) und eine erfolgreiche akademische Laufbahn (Duncan et
al., 2007). Allerdings lernt nicht jedes Kind lesen, schreiben
und rechnen mit der gleichen Leichtigkeit (M. Brown et al.,
2003; Cockcroft, 1982). Darüber hinaus sind die neuralen Ursprünge individueller Unterschiede in solch komplexen kognitiven Fähigkeiten noch immer umstritten.

Die Erforschung spezifischer neuraler Korrelate der Lese-,
Schreib- und Rechenkompetenz steht besonderen Heraus-
forderungen gegenüber. Erstens sind Längsschnittstudien erforderlich, die mit der Erhebung bereits vor Schuleintritt begin-
nen und so neurobiologische Profile und Entwicklungsverläufe
identifizieren können, die im direkten Zusammenhang mit Ver-
haltensvielfalt stehen (Goswami, 2015; Ramus et al., 2018). Bis-
lang sind solche längsschnittlichen Betrachtungen jedoch selten.
Zweitens muss die beträchtliche Kovariation zwischen Lese-,
Schreib- und Rechenleistungen (Durand et al., 2005; Hart et

al., 2009) bei der Erforschung spezifischer Korrelate einzelner Fähigkeiten berücksichtigt werden. Drittens ist möglicherweise eine ganzheitlichere Vorgehensweise vonnöten, die mehrere anatomische und funktionale Dimensionen kombiniert und so ein umfassenderes Verständnis der Entstehung komplexer kognitiver Fähigkeiten und ihrer Entwicklungsverläufe bietet.

Das Ziel der vorliegenden Arbeit war es, einen Einblick in neurale Entwicklungsverläufe zu gewinnen, die den initialen Erwerb von Lese-, Schreib- und Rechenkompetenz unterstützen. Dazu haben wir die die Zusammenhänge von Gehirn und komplexen kognitiven Fähigkeiten mittels struktureller und funktioneller Magnetresonanztomografie im Ruhezustand untersucht. Die vorliegenden Studien kombinieren Analysen längsschnittlicher Bildgebungsdaten von Kindern, die am Ende der Kindergartenzeit und im Schulalter erhoben wurden, mit umfangreichen psychometrischen Tests. Dabei konzentriert sich diese Arbeit auf zwei Kernfragen: Was sind neurale Korrelate von (a) defizitärem Schriftspracherwerb und (b) individuellen Unterschieden in der Entwicklung mathematischer Fähigkeiten? Die längsschnittliche Betrachtung dieser Fragen offenbarte spezifische neurale Profile, die in Zusammenhang mit phänotypischer Verhaltensvariation stehen. Im Einzelnen quantifizierten die vorgestellten Analysen unterschiedliche neuroanatomische und -funktionale Maße, während für relevante Kovariate wie dem soziodemographischen Status, intellektuellen Fähigkeiten und individueller Lese-, Schreib- und Rechenleistung kontrolliert wurde.

In der ersten vorliegenden Studie wurde systematisch untersucht, ob wissenschaftliche Theorien zur Entstehung von Legasthenie potentielle entwicklungsbedingte Ursachen oder eher Folgen der reduzierten Übung im Umgang mit Schriftsprache beschreiben. In der Tat existieren diverse Ansichten, die verschiedene neurobiologische Ursprünge spezifischer Defizite im Schriftspracherwerb nahelegen. Diese reichen von Beeinträchtigungen auditorischer (Díaz et al., 2012; Hornickel & Kraus, 2013) oder visueller (Eden et al., 1996; Livingstone et al., 1991) Signalwege, über generelle, magnozelluläre Störungen (Stein, 2001; Stein & Walsh, 1997) und Theorien zerebellarer Defizite (Nicolson et al., 2001), bis hin zu Fehlleistungen innerhalb übergeordneter Prozesse im phonologischen Sprachverarbeitungssystem (Boets et al., 2013; S. E. Shaywitz et al., 1998). Problematisch ist jedoch, dass diese Theorien in erster Linie auf Erkenntnissen von Untersuchungen in Erwachsenen oder Schulkindern beruhen. Daher kann nicht ausgeschlossen werden, dass Unterschiede zwischen Legasthenie- und Kontrollgruppen durch einen abweichenden Umgang mit Schriftsprache getrieben werden (Goswami, 2015; Ramus et al., 2018). Um dieses Problem zu umgehen, wurden hier Messungen der funktionellen Magnetresonanztomographie im Ruhezustand, der T_1- und der Diffusions-gewichteten Bildgebung in Kindern vor und nach Beginn der formalen Schriftsprachanleitung in der Schule erhoben. 16 Kinder wurden auf der Grundlage standardisierter Lese- und Reschtschreibtests im Schulalter als legasthenisch eingestuft und mit 16 Kindern ohne Auffälligkeiten im Schriftspracherwerb verglichen. Im Einzelnen wurden strukturelle und funktionelle Maße komplexer kortikaler und sub-kortikaler Netzwerke, die zuvor mit Legasthenie in Verbindung gebracht wurden, zwischen beiden Gruppen verglichen.

Die Ergebnisse zeigen einen Zusammenhang zwischen dem Auftreten von Legasthenie, kortikalen Fehlbildungen und reduzierter funktioneller Konnektivität innerhalb des Sprachverarbeitungssystems. Im Einzelnen zeigte sich bei Kindern mit zukünftigen Problemen im Schriftspracherwerb ein höherer Grad kortikaler Faltung vor und nach Beginn der formalen Schriftsprachanleitung in der Schule. Außerdem haben wir vorübergehende Unterschiede in der strukturellen und funktionellen Konnektivität linkshemipsherischer, perisylvischer Regionen beobachtet. Diese umfassten eine stärkere Konnektivität zwischen dem Planum Temporale und dem Brodmann-

Areal 6 durch den Fasciculus Arcuatus und reduzierte funktionelle Konnektivität zwischen dem primären auditorischen Kortex und dem Planum Temporale. Vorhersagemodelle, die auf diese Ergebnisse aufbauen, zeigten allein und in Kombination mit relevanten Verhaltensmaßen statistisch signifikante Klassifikationsraten. Diese Befunde erweitern die bisher spärliche empirische Evidenz neuroanatomischer Auffälligkeiten innerhalb des Sprachverarbeitungssystems in Kindern mit Problemen im Schriftspracherwerb vor Eintritt in die Schule (Clark et al., 2014). Dadurch unterstützen die vorliegenden Ergebnisse Theorien, die Legasthenie ein spezifisches phonologisches Defizit zugrunde legen. Dieses bedingt möglicherweise geringere phonologische Fähigkeiten, die wiederum den Aufbau zuverlässiger Assoziationen zwischen Buchstaben und den zugehörigen Lauten stören (Snowling, 1998). Auf dieser Grundlage schlage ich vor, dass atypische kortikale Faltung der primären Hörrinde und gestörte funktionelle Konnektivität zwischen perisylvischen Regionen möglicherweise als Konsequenz abweichender neuronaler Migration entstehen. Die Unterschiede in der Faserstärke des Fasciculus Arcuatus könnten so als Folge des Einsatzes artikulatorischer Kompensationsstrategien, die durch den ventralen prämotorischen Kortex unterstützt werden (Pugh et al., 2000; Richlan et al., 2011; S. E. Shaywitz et al., 1998) entstehen. Eine solches

Szenario muss in Folgestudien konkretisiert werden. Zudem sind weitere Studien notwendig, um die vorliegenden Ergebnisse zu validieren und deren Generalisierbarkeit auch auf andere, nicht-alphabetische oder weniger transparente Schriftsysteme zu untersuchen.

In der zweiten Studie haben wir den Zusammenhang zwischen kortikaler Plastizität vom letzten Kindergartenjahr an bis hin zur zweiten Klasse und der individuellen Leistung in arithmetischer und visuell-räumlicher Mengenverarbeitung untersucht. Zu diesem Zweck wurden Daten von 28 Kindern ohne Lernentwicklungsstörungen längsschnittlich ausgewertet. Hinweise für die Rolle struktureller und funktioneller Plastizität in Kernregionen der Mengenverarbeitung im rechten posterioren parietalen Kortex für die verhaltenstypische Entwicklung von Rechenfähigkeiten finden sich in der Literatur (Cantlon et al., 2006; Menon, 2010; Rivera et al., 2005). Zusätzlich gibt es Belege für die Einbeziehung von Regionen, die typischerweise mit Arbeitsgedächtnis- und Aufmerksamkeitsprozessen verbunden werden, bei noch nicht voll ausgereifter mathematischer Verarbeitung (i. e. präfrontale Areale; Rivera et al., 2005). Mit steigendem Alter und mathematischer Übung verringert sich der Beitrag dieser Prozesse für numerische Kognition, während die funktionelle Spezialisierung des linken posterioren parietalen Kortex voranschreitet (Rivera et al., 2005). Die zusätzliche Beteiligung des medialen Schläfenlappens für die Entwicklung mathematischer Verarbeitung weist zudem auf die Bildung und Konsolidierung gedächtnisbasierter Strategien für mathematisches Problemlösen hin (Qin et al., 2014).

Die Ergebnisse der zweiten Studie zeigen Verbindungen zwischen früher arithmetischer und visuell-räumlicher Mengenverarbeitung—zwei Grundkompetenzen numerischer Fähigkeiten—und kortikaler Reorganisation innerhalb rechtshemisphärischer Areale. Im Einzelnen korrelierten arithmetische Fähigkeiten signifikant mit Plastizität kortikaler Faltung des rechten Sulcus intraparietalis und kortikaler Dicke der Spitze des Temporallappens. Gleichzeitig haben wir gezeigt, dass visuell-räumliche Mengenverarbeitung signifikant mit Veränderungen der kortikalen Dicke im Lobulus parietalis superior und im Gyrus praecentralis, sowie mit Plastizität der kortikalen Faltung im mittleren Teil des Frontallappens zusammenhängt. Somit legen unsere Ergebnisse eine Aufteilung des Parietallappens in den Sulcus intraparietalis als domänenspezifisches Zentrum der neurale Repräsentationen von Zahlen und Mengen, und dem Lobulus parietalis superior als ein Areal, das die visuell-räumliche Ausrichtung von Aufmerksamkeit unterstützt, nahe (Dehaene et al., 2003). Des Weiteren stimmen die Befunde in Regionen, die mit Prozessen des Arbeitsgedächtnisses verbunden sind, mit vorangegangenen Studien überein, die zeigten, dass die Arbeitsgedächtnisleistung einen wesentlichen Teil der behavioralen Varianz in mathematischen Aufgaben erklärt (Raghubar et al., 2010). Angesichts der ausschließlich rechts-hemisphärischen Befunde schlage ich vor, dass rechtsseitige Prozesse im Besonderen die initiale Entwicklung von Rechenkompetenzen unterstützen. Daraus folgt die Hypothese, dass linksseitige Befunde, wie in Studien mit Schulkindern gezeigt (Rivera et al., 2005), durch spätere Übung mit und Reifung von mathematischen Prozessen entstehen. Dies könnte Untersuchungsgegenstand zukünftiger Studien sein.

Insgesamt beleuchtet die vorliegende Arbeit Entwicklungsverläufe, die dem Erwerb von Schriftsprach- und Rechenkompetenz zugrunde liegen. Somit stellen die Befunde einen wesentlichen Schritt in Richtung eines umfassenderen Verständnisses der Entstehung komplexer kognitiver Fähigkeiten und spezifischer Fehlentwicklungen, die möglicherweise Lernstörungen hervorrufen, dar. Zum einen legen die vorliegenden Ergebnisse nahe, dass der Erwerb und die Entwicklung komplexer Fähigkeiten mit Plastizität von Netzwerken im Gehirn zusammenhängen, die domänenspezifische sowie domänenübergreifende Funktionen unterstützen (z.B. Mengen-, visuell-räumliche und Arbeitsgedächtnisprozesse für Rechenkompetenz). Zum anderen

deuten sie darauf hin, dass Störungen in Regionen, die sehr spez-

ifische Aspekte komplexer kognitiver Fähigkeiten unterstützen,

schwerwiegende Konsequenzen für den Erwerb haben kön-

nen (z.B. eine Beeinträchtigung der phonologischen Sprachver-

arbeitung, die den Schriftspracherwerb behindert).

DECLARATION

I, Ulrike Kuhl, hereby confirm that this thesis entitled "The brain basis of emerging literacy and numeracy skills – Longitudinal neuroimaging evidence from kindergarten to primary school" is my own original work. Auxiliary sources and work of others that I used has been acknowledged. I have not made use of any other resources or means than those indicated.

Ich, Ulrike Kuhl, bestätige hiermit die hier vorliegende Arbeit mit dem Titel „The brain basis of emerging literacy and numeracy skills – Longitudinal neuroimaging evidence from kindergarten to primary school" selbstständig verfasst zu haben. Andere Werke und Quellen auf die ich mich beziehe, habe ich kenntlich gemacht. Ich habe keine anderen Hilfsmittel als die angegebenen verwendet.

Leipzig, 18.03.2019

Ulrike Kuhl

MPI Series in Human Cognitive and Brain Sciences:

mit dem Effekt jener Fitness, die erforderlich ist, um unter den gegebenen Rahmenbedingungen bestehen zu können. Zum anderen gibt es aber auch die Anpassung der Umwelt an den Menschen – wir nennen dies dann Kultur. In beiden Fällen führt die konsequente Negierung der erforderlichen Anpassungsmechanismen das Individuum und letztendlich auch das Kollektiv ins Verderben.

Speisereste greifen. Und es könnte sein, dass Sie einen Döner oder Hotdog essenden Jugendlichen dabei beobachten, wie er seine Finger an der Sitzbank reinigt, und wenn Sie ihn darauf ansprechen, im besten Fall einen mitleidigen Blick begleitet von einem leisen Schulterzucken als Antwort bekommen. Es könnte aber auch sein, dass Sie folgende Antwort bekommen: „Was geht Sie das an – gehört die Bank Ihnen?" Sie könnten aber auch jener Kundin begegnet sein, die im Supermarkt aus dem Kühlregal eine Packung Fischstäbchen nahm, es sich dann anders überlegte und diese nicht, wie man annehmen möchte, wieder dort deponierte, sondern ganz ungeniert in das für Frischgebäck vorgesehene Regal legte. Eine andere Kundin, die dies sah, sprach die Dame auf ihr Fehlverhalten an und bekam eine ganz klare Botschaft mit auf den Weg: „Kümmern Sie sich um Ihren eigenen […] – und wenn Ihnen das so wichtig ist, dann tragen Sie es selbst zurück!"

Ich habe die Erlebnisse und Beobachtungen, die ich im Rahmen von Gesprächen mit mehr oder minder betroffenen Personen erfahren durfte, natürlich nur exemplarisch wiedergegeben. Aber ich hoffe, ich konnte damit aufzeigen, dass es gegenwärtig bei bestimmten Zeitgenossen unschicklich (im Sinne von unzeitgemäß) sein kann, jene Verhaltensweisen einzufordern, die getragen sind von Verantwortung, gepflegten Umgangsformen, Respekt und Höflichkeit und die man bis dato unter dem Begriff „zivilisiertes Benehmen" subsumiert hatte.

Ich denke, wir müssten uns wieder jene grundlegende anthropologische Erkenntnis bewusst vor Augen führen, dass unserer Entfaltung bzw. Menschwerdung zwei entscheidende Entwicklungen vorangegangen sind, die bekanntermaßen ja auch noch andauern: zum einen die Evolution, also die Anpassung des Menschen an seine jeweiligen Umweltbedingungen gende Formalismen" handelt, sondern um einen unverzichtbaren gemeinnützigen Stabilitätsfaktor, der der gegenwärtig ansteigenden Geringschätzung Menschen und Dingen gegenüber Einhalt gebieten könnte.

Ordnungen wie ein demokratisches Rechtssystem, die Sprache, die Gestalt einer auf die Bedürfnisse der Bewohner ausgerichteten Stadt, die Gliederung eines Tages, das gesittete Einnehmen einer Mahlzeit und grundlegende Formen der Höflichkeit möchte ich hier – wenn auch nur bruchstückhaft – ansprechen.

Ich kann mich nämlich zuweilen des Eindrucks nicht erwehren, dass grundlegend zivilisiertes Verhalten oder das Einfordern desselben immer öfter als anstößig empfunden wird. Da wird mit dem Handy bzw. Smartphone in Arztpraxen und Restaurants ungeniert telefoniert, da werden teilweise intime oder dem Datenschutz unterliegende Informationen lautstark allen anderen Anwesenden mitgeteilt, ohne Rücksicht, ob die daran interessiert sind oder nicht. Und sollten Sie glauben, wenn Sie die telefonierende Person darauf ansprechen, dass diese ihr Gespräch dann unterbricht oder gar beendet, dann haben Sie sich in den meisten Fällen getäuscht (Ausnahmen bestätigen natürlich den Regelfall). Nein, er oder sie sieht Sie an, als hätten Sie nicht alle Sinne beisammen.

Allerdings konnte ich in einer Arztpraxis beobachten, dass eine Patientin, die nach einem zehnminütigen Gespräch die Deutschschularbeit ihres Sohnes betreffend von der Sprechstundenhilfe höflich aufgefordert wurde, das Gespräch zu beenden, die Praxis mit folgenden (ihrer Gesprächspartnerin Gertrude zugewandten) Worten verließ: „Du, wart ein bisserl, ich geh raus, die da regt sich auf!"

Es kann Ihnen aber auch passieren, dass Sie in einem öffentlichen Verkehrsmittel in eine Halteschlaufe greifen und zu spät bemerken, dass Sie in Reste von Ketchup oder andere cremige